CHANNELING
THE
WHISPERS WITHIN

A SCHIZOPHRENIC'S JOURNEY
Through the Labyrinth of Life

CHANNELING
THE
WHISPERS WITHIN

A SCHIZOPHRENIC'S JOURNEY
Through the Labyrinth of Life

Timothy V. Lane

Third Eye Publishing
Red Oak, Texas

CHANNELING
THE
WHISPERS WITHIN
A SCHIZOPHRENIC'S JOURNEY
Through the Labyrinth of Life

Published by
Third Eye Book Publishing
Red Oak, Texas

voncewaylon@gmail.com

Timothy Lane, President, Co-CEO and Publisher
Mahogany Byrd Co-CEO, Associate Publisher
Zharia Ransom Editor/Editorial Director
Yvonne Rose/Quality Press.info, Book Packager

Dedication

This book is dedicated to my Parents; both sets of Grandparents; my aunts and uncles; my sister; my Beautiful Queen, Mahogany, and our kids; my nieces, nephews, and a whole host of cousins. But probably just as important, I dedicate this book to my doctors, Dr. Inna Kogan (Psychiatry) and Dr. Jeffrey Thompson (Dallas Kidney Specialist) who worked together and discovered a link between kidney disease (Lupus Nephritis) and Schizophrenia. Due to their excellent expertise in their respective fields, I am able to show in this book that I am a product of good doctors and just delightful human beings who really care about the people they treat. To them I want to say "thank you" from the bottom of my heart. I would not be here if it were not for you, and everyone mentioned in this dedication.

Third Eye Publishing

Acknowledgments

I would like to acknowledge:

Dr. Booker T, Bobby Hemmitt, Phil Valentine, Dr. John L. Johnson, and Jay Chang.

The Hebrew Israelites, and ancient Ethiopian and Egyptian culture and theology.

Also, a special acknowledgement to our people.

Third Eye Publishing

Contents

Third Eye Publishing

Introduction

Hello, I am Timothy V. Lane. If you have read my first book, then you know that I suffer from what is known as paranoid Schizophrenia. Though now that it is more commonly known, I still, believe it or not, come across some people who do not know what Schizophrenia is. They have no idea. So, for those of you who are interested, let me explain the dynamics of this condition.

As explained from the American Psyche Association, Schizophrenia is a chronic brain disorder that affects less than one percent of the U.S. population. When it is active, symptoms can include delusions, hallucinations, disorganized speech, trouble with thinking, and lack of motivation. While there is no cure for Schizophrenia, research is leading to innovative and safer treatments.

Experts are also unraveling the causes of the disease by studying genetics, conducting research, and using advanced imaging to look at the brain structure and function. These approaches hold the promise of new, and more effective therapies. The complexity of Schizophrenia may help explain why there are misconceptions about the disease.

Schizophrenia does not mean split personality or multiple personality disorder. Most people with Schizophrenia are not any more dangerous or violent than people in the general population. While limited mental health resources in the community may lead to homelessness and frequent hospitalization, it is a misconception that people with Schizophrenia end up homeless or living in hospitals. Most live with their family, in group homes, or on their own.

When the disease is active it can be characterized by episodes where the person is unable to distinguish between real and unreal experiences. As with any illness, the severity, duration, and frequency of symptoms can vary; however, in persons with Schizophrenia, the incidence of severe psychotic symptoms often decreases as the person becomes older. Not taking medications as prescribed, the use of alcohol or illicit drugs, and stressful situations tend to lead to increased symptoms.

PART I

What Drove Me Insane

Third Eye Publishing

A MORE IN-DEPTH LOOK: ZHARIA

People who suffer from Schizophrenia are what I consider special. I have audio and visual hallucinations, which means I hear voices and see things, visions, if you will. I think people who suffer from this illness can tap into a part of their brain that most others cannot. These people are able to use more than 10% of their brain capacity. We see things differently, leading up to ultimately doing things differently. We are trapped inside of our minds, trying to escape the prison and get the message out. The message to me is that nothing appears to be what it seems. It seems as if there is good and evil, but that is just a microcosm of what we have become as creators, really, we are just soul and flesh, positive and negative charges.

It seems as if it is a battle, but really it is just a balancing act of the two teetering on the scales of consciousness, existence, and material. As I stated in my last publication, everything has opposites. Those opposites feed and feed off each other. You would not know what light is unless you have been in the dark. You would not know of negative energy unless you had experienced positive energy. You would not know what good is unless you have faced evil.

Your flesh would not recognize your soul unless it was somehow connected through this embodiment of structure that we exist in; everything coinciding together and ultimately, the ultimate opposite; Man would not know himself if it was not for the woman, and vice versa. My problem for the longest time was that I was not surrounded by like minds. Most of my peers were lost in ignorance. So, I felt alone for the better part of 25 years. I always said that the only thing scarier than being blind is being the only one who can see. It drove me even crazier, because no one could see what I see or hear what I hear. I became angry and secluded, isolated within myself. Someone eventually came to my aide. *Her name shall remain anonymous.* Anyway, when I was first diagnosed with this disease, I had a friend of the family who would call and check on me.

I was living with my grandparents then. She called me one day and we started talking. I told her that I was searching for a certain female that I remembered from my childhood pre-k class. Her name was Heaven Star (first and middle name). I remembered how she looked back then as a child. She had blue eyes. Well, my friend who shall remain anonymous told me that she, herself, had a cousin named Heaven Star. I immediately thought that this was the girl I was searching for. However, the Heaven Star I was looking for graduated from Dallas David W. Carter High School in 1996. This Heaven Star graduated from the rival Dallas Justin F. Kimball high school in 1996. To be sure that this was not the girl that I was looking for, I asked my friend what color her eyes were, and she said green. Go figure that, blue and green.

I was starting to believe I had the world within my reach. Remembering opposites, at that time (1998-1999), I was searching for the kingdom of heaven. I was channeling my energy into two representations of the kingdom, these two heavens, these two beautiful African American women, soul, and flesh. Suddenly, I was viewing the world differently. I was not sexually, but spiritually intimate with those two worlds. One became my life, and the other was my afterlife, both developing together at the same time. I told my anonymous friend that her cousin was not the one I was looking for. But I was still curious about what this could mean. I felt one with my father, and my mother was as nurturing as the holy spirit. I was already feeling like I might be the Messiah anyway. If you read my first book, then you know why I was feeling that way.

Not to say that I was, but I was three things that white Amerikkka was afraid of, young, black, and confident. Now, only if I could just use my love for the heavens to influence the rest of my people to feel this way. It became a must. If this is what it seems, then the goal is to set up the kingdom of heaven on Earth. Then the heavens and I would give God the glory (God being the absolute; the Black family).

Now, some of you may believe in the messiah, on the contrary, others may not. No matter what side of the spectrum you are on, it is believed that the darker complected people need something or someone powerful to organize a plan to put our people back in positions of power on this planet. They tell us that we are the minority. But the reality is that there are 7.5 billion people on the planet. Eighty-five percent of those people are people of color or of African descent. So how is it that the vast majority of the people who are on this planet are the ones being oppressed?

All it takes is education and a desire to want to improve our conditions. We can seize control by force if we all unite. These are things and issues I would bring up when talking to the heavens. I figured and felt like it was up to the three of us. For me, their fleshly passions were fueling me to carry out the plan. I could feel it. I could feel their passion. It gave them focus and made them stronger. It gave them focus to the point to where they are so locked in on the process of creation; And what I was attempting to do with them was to create. At that time, there were no physical conversations, for I was hearing their voices, and I would speak back to them. I was conversing with them on a whole other level. I was using telepathy. Inside my mind and all around my being, there are seven voices that I am loyal to, seven family members, including my mother. Those seven voices are angels to me. My seven stars, which illuminate my being. There are seven letters in the word heavens.

As far as I was concerned, I was communicating with them and getting them to a point of comfort by introducing to them the art of feeding off of their lust and their needs by tempting them with their wants. What they wanted was a king, what they needed to raise and move the spirits within them was a God. Global warming intensified in 1998 and up until now, because of the spiritual, sexual, and intimate pressure I have been placing on the heavens to stay connected to me, I was intimate with them spiritually before it manifested physically.

Really, when this all began, I was on a quest to find God and I found them, like minds. I was more attracted to their minds. I wanted to erase everything that we were taught through religion and what we learned in school and bring a new knowledge of self, a higher self and higher intelligence. I was vibrating on a different frequency, and I needed them to vibrate with me. All I ever wanted them to do was live up to their name. I, at least, was trying to live up to mine.

My initials are T.V.L. The TV part of my name was sort of a spin-off of the initials "TV," or television (tell a vision). I was that for so long and in some ways I still am. My late grandfather used to say that the T.V. was the most evil of all things that can generate a frequency... I guess because of the psychological effects of programming and imaging. Nevertheless, in some instances, this became me and in certain cases, I was just as entertaining as a television to most people. Listening to me talk, the things that I would talk about were like a live show to most people, when I was younger, before the dark times. I was trying to live up to more than just my initials though.

When I was first stricken with Schizophrenia, the first time that I heard voices, I was reading the book of Revelations. Then somewhere around Revelations chapters 19 and 20, I was convinced and confident that the voices were coming from me, but also surrounding me. There were seven family members, four aunts, two uncles and one cousin, (the eldest of my grandmother's grandchildren). All of these people were alive, or shall I say on this side when I first experienced this. That is why it was so strange.

I reached out to a Christian preacher, and he told me he could understand how I could be hearing the dead, but what was puzzling to him was that he could not understand how I could be hearing the living. He told me that he was not qualified to deal with a matter such as mine. Anyway, the voices were telling me that I was God. Then they would say that I was the devil or the antichrist. Then some of them would tell me that I am Jesus or the Messiah. All of this was confusing to me, and I became angry.

Then I heard a woman's voice. The voice spoke to me and said that she was heaven. She told me she was with me and that I am nothing more than what I am. That was significant because what I learned is that the "I am" is eternal, the Elohim, or Eloham, the yin and the yang, the atom or star, or Adam. The am means lord; And I can say that I am, and the female entity or being is her, Heaven. Matter or material was meant to be molded into existence from my word. My dilemma was that I was interacting with these two females intimately or spiritually, not physically. It was sort of like an intimate telepathy, they were there but they were not there. I had not even run into them physically; I just knew that they were alive and that they were with me.

But which one of them was speaking to me inside my mind? I could not tell. When I would ask the spirit, everything in my mind went quiet. Anyway, with all that I was learning about the Amen-Ra or the Atom-Ra and reinventing myself, and my cause for being here, I aimed at educating them with this new knowledge of self, Blackness, and black thought. I was trying to erase the European brainwashing that went on for centuries, clean out of our spiritual and physical systems. (Revelations.21:3) "Then I saw a new heaven and a new Earth, for the first heaven and the first earth had passed away, and there was no longer any sea. I saw the holy city, the new Jerusalem coming down out of Heaven from God prepared as a bride beautifully dressed for her husband."

I was trying to transform them into something greater, make them new, show them how to build wealth and generate and get lost in the anticipation of an orgasm whether it be mental, spiritual, or physical, clitoral or vaginal. I wanted them to have a sense of self-worth. What better way to do that than to show them all of this that I was experiencing and the vision I had for the people all over the world, Black supremacy, to be one with God as I was one with the Heavens and the voices.

The voices represent the ancestors and multitudes of Black people. Whether or not you think that the book of Revelations is legit in history or not, some spirit used that book to get my attention and now even if you don't believe in a Messiah or that one ever walked the earth, now, in 1978 a way was made for one to come through into existence. The goal was to place blackness back on top where it belongs. To do this, we have to think that we are, as in, we are the stars. The beast 666, 6 electrons, 6 neutrons, 6 protons, the makeup of the carbon atom or Adam. The Amen (as it is called by the ancient Babylonians and Hebrews) is that. It is the makeup of the physical universe. The word Kemet also gave birth to the word chemical (kemical), and the universe is a combination of chemicals.

Trying to get people to understand this, as it applied to us, was driving me crazy. Trying to get the heavens to understand this was driving me insane. I quickly realized how lost we were. If the fate of the world was dependent on us, then we and everyone (Black people) were in trouble. We for generations and centuries looked for a white messiah to come down from the sky and save us. The reality, though, is that there is no Messiah, but us. We are the only saviors, Black people. Until we can curb our animalistic urges and behavior, and vibrate on a higher frequency, we will never reach a higher intelligence (God). Thus, we will become separated from the organic, or God, and dwell in a place of torment and nothing (Hell).

They say that God will put no more on you than you can bear. But this was a lot of weight to hold, to try to convince people that if they wanted to see God, then all they had to do was look in the mirror. Then on top of that I had to convince the lost heavens that I had not lost, let alone, I had to convince myself first. So here we are, confirmation. Confirmation in the sense that all that I was seeking, spiritually, started with me. I just looked inside and saw straight through into the heavens, no one but me. And so, I took the prize. The price that I paid was that I was indulged in an eternal fight to have joy and be confident. The situation was a little too hard to believe. To be frank, it seemed too good to be true.

There were these two. There are so many coincidences that connect Heaven Star, and Heaven Star and me together that to go through a few would be frightening. I felt like I had to be the Messiah, not for me, my family, or myself, but for the Heavens too. Then there were the people, people who believed so hard in a savior, a savior who could not see any other way out but through these two heavens. Educating the people on our history and connection to the stars and the universe. For that is something in which we were taught and thought to be evil.

But the study of alchemy is the study of melanin. The fact that melanin at the height of its power is plasma, blood, black blood. It is the darkness of the universe, and it (melanin) cannot be controlled, contained, or corralled and that is frightening to the European race. I needed to get everyone on the same page. I needed my people to stop giving all their energy to a god that has no power. Jezeus (Jesus) Zeus never existed as a physical being because Greek mythology is derived from Egyptian mythology. In Greek mythology, Zeus, king of the gods, is the equivalent of Amen-ra, the Egyptian king of the gods. The Am in amen is significant. Zeus, Jezeus is imaginary. I can say that I AM.

We are taught that melanin is evil in reality, it is omnipotent and essential to the beauty and power which is the universe. It is what makes us who we are. We walk differently, we talk differently, we have rhythm in our makeup and aura, which allows our bodies to communicate through the soul. Telepathy is how I've been communicating with the heavens. Though not together physically, we are connected through the great cerebral connection that connects and binds all living things inside this energy field that we call life. Through this connection, I can speak directly to them about them, and for them; and everything inside and around them will listen and be affected, just as I was when the seven spirits spoke to me.

Though my people continue to fall by the wayside, I consider myself more blessed than cursed. These things that I have described to you are part of the blessing that is in store for all of us. The curse does not have anything to do with our oppressors. The curse has everything to do with the fact that knowledge, wisdom, and power are right in front of us now. But because we are ignorant and oppress ourselves by purposely not recognizing it, we cannot seem to free ourselves; whether it comes from our oppressors, or our own consciences and imaginations molded by our oppressors.

As I stated in my first book, every element found in the known universe is in each star in the universe. Each element found in the universe and space is also found in humanity. I emphasize the word hue because the first homo-sapien was a melanated human, the scripture tells us his name is Adam. I, as I understand things inside my schizophrenic mind, correlate the father Adam with the scientific Atom, which is the basic building block of nature, being that Adam or Atom was created from cosmic dust. I have always thought that we are not separate from the organic (of God). The atom or Adam is the light or the star. Light is heat and energy, energy is life.

In my research, I found a notable source (s). Mr. John L. Johnson, wrote the book, "The Black Biblical History: 4000 Years of Black History, vol. 16." In that book, he was mentioning some of the most ancient names for God, and amen- RA (chief Egyptian deity) was also called Atum- RA or Atom- RA. He (Mr. Johnson) also had more sources to prove this in that book. Among some of the other things that I learned from him was that the name or word Adam means

15

GOD. If all of this were true, this would place the beginnings of the Black man back as far as not only to the beginning of the world but to the very beginning and creation of the universe.

PART II

Waking From the Dead

Third Eye Publishing

TIMILLE

With all of this being the case, how have we as a race fallen to the bottom and depths of society? Now I struggle with taking my medicine, but how do I know if these medicines are designed to control the way that I think or feel?

What if they are designed to suppress the most potent of my emotions which is my confidence? Look, it's no secret that many of the European race will go to extraordinary lengths to discredit or even kill the Blacks. I just assume that the reason for the genocide and massacres is because the Europeans know what kind of power we hold. The problem is that we don't know. So, my goal became to educate our people on the origins and powers of melanin and our pineal gland because it looks as if that may be the key and the only thing that will save us.

Not only that, but we need to find ways to accumulate wealth, enough wealth to circulate back to Black communities. We need to have Black Wall Streets all over America, along with our own militias to protect our properties and people from white supremacists and radical, racial extremists. Really, everything is about energy. What you put out, you will receive. As pertaining to white supremacists, the energy that has been produced by them is negative; filled with hatred, jealousy, and envy.

For 2500 years or more, melanated people have produced an energy of substance, because of enslavement. Nonetheless, we suffered a great deal at the hands of our own race, the Arab race, and the European race through the Trans- Atlantic Slave Trade, which actually began after 70 A.D. (C.E). We still as a race contributed more than a lion's share to society in the fields of mathematics, science, agriculture, economics, and religion. The origins of Judaism, Islam, and Christianity lie with Black people and our connection to the stars and the universe. The universe is filled with energy (or stars and planets).

We have a soul, which comprises of seven energy centers inside the human body that directly connect us to the cosmos. These energy centers are called chakras, seven cycling, circling energy centers in the body that move like solar systems around galaxies. These are wheels of light inside the human body, inner suns as I call them. This is some valuable information from something I studied on the Chakra System. Chakras and Black people, it's not spooky, but rather more relevant than religion. The chakra system is about learning who you are and understanding your body and its energy based on its understanding as it relates to the cosmos.

The seven chakras, as explained, can help with self-understanding and the quest is to know thyself. Learning all that you can possibly know about yourself is important. The chakra system is intended specifically for you to learn yourself and become aware of who you are and your actions.

1st: The root chakra (red) usually called the first chakra, is the lowest of the seven-chakra system and the most basic of them all. Survival, sexuality, stability, and sensuality, this is how we form relationships and bonds in modern society and culture. Being aware of your sexuality helps in choosing a suitable mate for survival. We want to pass down as much duplication as possible. The color red is always associated with the chakra, the Muladhara, and is used to focus or channel the body's energy into stimulating these specific functions. Hematite is the stone associated with the root chakra and is supposed to help with meditation and balance of this specific chakra system.

2nd: The sacral chakra or second chakra is known as the source chakra for reproduction. It is the chakra of the testes and the ovaries. The second chakra encompasses traits that we find ourselves practicing like violence, addictions, basic emotional needs, and pleasure. We must remember that all are connected. Just as this chakra can govern bad traits, it can also govern good ones like joy, enthusiasm, and creativity. Carnelian is the stone associated with the sacral chakra; if you are attempting to bear children this stone is helpful to have around the house or in the room you tend to conceive in. (orange)

3rd: The third chakra, the solar plexus is the chakra that is the belly of the beast. It is the digestive system. They say you are what you eat; this is the reason. The solar plexus is fed by the sun, and foods that feed off the sunlight do well to help cultivate the elevation of this chakra. As with all the chakras, certain emotions or characteristics are associated with the third chakra. This includes personal power, fear, anxiety, opinion formation, introversion, and transition from simple emotions to complex ones. The third chakra is associated with mental expansion, the Manipura, or your growth chakra. The stone associated with the third chakra is citrine and should be kept in your kitchen while you are preparing meals. (gold)

4th: The fourth chakra, the heart, the center of it all, is one of the most important things to focus on. The symbol for the heart chakra is familiar as well as the color. If you are familiar with Egyptian spiritual knowledge, you understand as above; so below, if you look into the symbol, you will notice two pyramids - one right side up and one upside down. This symbolizes you, your upper and lower self. As we begin to go through the upper chakras you begin to see the higher realm of thought and emotions concerning each. The heart chakra is your center. The fourth chakra or Anahata-puri is the healing factor of the chakra system. It is associated with the development of resistance to outside attacks. This chakra is the key to the next life. Purity of the heart is important; compassion, tenderness, unconditional love, equilibrium, rejection & well-being, are all associated with the heart chakra, and the most important is passion. Rose Quartz is the stone associated with the heart chakra and if possible, should be incorporated into a necklace with gold as the primary conductor to the body. (Green)

5th: The fifth chakra, the throat, is stimulated a lot daily as the sky is blue and resonates with us frequently. Communication is the realm of the fifth chakra. With clear focus, you can channel the fifth chakra to understand your thoughts and move them more frequently up the chakra system. The fifth chakra is a projection of your self-confidence. The fifth chakra is what others encounter when having a conversation with you. The stone associated with the fifth chakra is sodalite, and whenever you feel you lack the confidence to speak the ideas it is the stone that should help your focus; or help you to focus on your chakra. (Blue)

6th: The sixth chakra, or the third eye Ajna is your gut feeling, your intuition, your third eye is what happens when you read between the lines and find the truth. Stimulation of the sixth chakra can be spiritual in feeling and unbelievable in reality. Those times that you felt like you should have gone with your gut feeling- that was your third eye activating, telling you which direction to go. The sixth chakra operates on the famine principle. The pineal gland is the sixth chakra location. Our brains are electric and should be fed oxygen as often as possible. Stimulating the sixth chakra can be done by simple tactics, magnets on your forehead or just eating electronic foods that contain zinc, copper, chromium, and even gold. The sixth chakra is important, so take good care to enhance it. The color for this chakra is indigo.

7th: The seventh chakra is the completion of the conscious, the center of your higher self. The seventh chakra is said to encompass your entire central nervous system and is said to also be connected to pineal and the pituitary gland, which ironically matches the Egyptian eye of Horus through an x-ray of the human brain. (image) *What did the ancients know?* The stone to enhance your connection to the seventh chakra is the Clear Quartz and this realm is pure belief and understanding of yourself, your consciousness, and your purpose. We are in control of ourselves and can focus on the many parts of our bodies that help us to form a complete understanding of self. The more you feel the need to study the chakra system, the more you're interested in knowing more about yourself. You choose to be at peace with your presence and adjust to the circumstances that encompass your life. The study of chakras is a resurging lifestyle, it is nonetheless, a rejection of modern religious corruption and the form of knowing yourself so that loving others won't be an issue."

The chakra system is karma; it is your energy. It is what you choose to be and live. Whether you know of your chakras or not, they are active. Universal Law is always active. Everything that you throw into the universe will come back to you so keep throwing positive energy out. The color for this chakra is purple or violet.

I want our people to know about how to enhance their melanin and ways to fully activate their pineal gland. I believe that melanin is tied directly to the chakras. Chakras are wheels of light and energy. Each of the seven main chakras is described as having a set number of "petals." When one adds the first six chakra petals, the sum becomes 144. The seventh chakra, or the crown chakra, which contains 1,000 petals, is then multiplied by the 144 sum which equals the product of 144,000. This number, 144,000, is synonymous with the speed of light. It is also biblically inclined. In the book of Revelations, chapter 14, it speaks of the 144,000 having the name of the lamb and the father's name written on their foreheads.

This is significant because the sixth chakra is the forehead and is where the pineal gland is located (also called the third eye). It goes on to say in the book of Revelations, chapter 14, verse three, "And they sang a new song before the throne and before the creatures and the elders." No one could learn the song except the 144,000 who had been redeemed from Earth. Now think about it, only one man, or shall I say, one being has been able to achieve this feat. You know him as Jesus, but as I explained earlier, Zeus never existed. We know from scripture that Christ (the Messiah) is a body (Body of Christ). We as believers make up the body of the Messiah. The question is what do we really believe? We know from science that the word

Christ is derivative of the word Cristos, which refers to the crystallization of stars, or what happens when melanin is compacted together; when blackness comes together; we explode and become pure light.

As you read this, I hope we have come to the realization that we, the Black man and woman, constitute the stars and space. So, either one man is going to reach that 144,000 chakra petals and become pure light or he and a certain number of people will achieve this feat, while still alive in the flesh. This makes me wonder if it is one or are we (his people) one. Not everyone is going to learn this knowledge, you are going to have some who are completely oblivious. "The 7 Stars that the Messiah (or the lamb, as he is called) holds in his right hand are the 7 chakras or 7 inner suns inside each individual human being; the 7 spirits of God as it is described in the book of Revelations.

Man is God and God is man; that's what I have come to believe, because we were created in God's image and likeness. We are the physical extension of the spiritual. They are thoughts; spirits, male and female manifested and embodied into the physical, which is us, the universe. The pre-fix, uni, means one, and Father God and mother nature, the male and female entity are one in us. Thus, in the scriptures, the Messiah refers to himself as "the son of man" because we created him. And now he is alive and breathing. God is light and light is energy and energy is life.

It is theorized that when all the chakras are vibrating and spinning at the appropriate rate, they produce an energy that becomes pure light. Thus, an individual becomes a light being or a light body. It has been alluded to earlier, that the pineal gland functions as a receiver for "energy" or "light." Thus, when the energy fields of the body are balanced harmoniously, the pineal gland reaches its optimum receptivity to universal energy. Once the chakras are balanced and attuned, an individual obtains "siddhis" or "supernatural" powers. With the pineal gland having such an increased sensitivity, the individual becomes "karast" or "anointed." We are inner-dimensional beings. No one can travel through space, because we are space, we are melanin. We are Israel and no man can get to the father (the riches, wealth, knowledge, and wisdom) unless they go through us. We are the energy, we are light, we are the way, both spiritually and scientifically.

Many African traditions, such as initiations, help to open the various chakra points in an individual's energy field. There have been many miraculous feats performed by African adepts that hold true to the sacred teachings of the ancestors. The Igbo Dibia is one such group of individuals. The various rituals inherent in our most ancient practices are done to concentrate energy. The old Per-Aa of ancient Kemet had the ritualized knowledge possessed by those master teachings. *Will this information be rediscovered if not already being put into practice presently?* When you start researching the chakra system, you will find a lot of information. Some of it will be conflicting and some of it will talk about what sort of experience you might have if you awaken the kundalini energy that is dormant at the base of your spine and start moving up through the chakra centers.

One post and source that I studied from a Yoga instructor makes a correlation between chakras and black holes. One commentary on the Bhagavad Gita talks about how Krishna and Arjuna are sitting in the middle of the battlefield. On the one side, which represents the ego, there is a tumultuous roar of noise before the battle. But on the other side that represents the soul, the warriors sound their instruments and there is a symphony of celestial sounds. These instruments represent the duality of the chaos of thinking on the ego's side versus the awakening of inner sound in different chakra centers during the depths of meditation on the soul's side. This actually is a good representation of the difference between the chakras' inner functioning and outer functioning, and how the psyche is connected to the universe. From her perspective, Chakras are like black holes… black holes form after the death of stars. They are massive holes in space that have such a dense amount of gravity that nothing that enters into them can escape from them. Not even particles of light. Black holes are mysteries. No one has been inside of one.

Scientists continue to speculate about their nature. But despite the mystery of what is contained inside of them, we can measure their effect on the space outside and around them. Black holes are such dense gravitational centers that everything in space revolves around them. Similarly, the moon revolves around the Earth, the Earth revolves around the sun, and the solar system revolves around a super massive black hole at the center of our galaxy. It seems to be a natural law that all things seek some center around which to gravitate and establish a rotational force.

This is probably one of Newton's laws. The Human body is not outside of these natural laws. Within the body, we have seven centers around which the physiological processes in the body revolve. Things like hormones and the spine and the heart and respiration and digestion and speech and thinking and elimination and reproduction and physical growth. Black holes form as a result of the death of stars. According to Wikipedia, "some primordial black holes could have formed at the beginning of the big bang and so they had a long time to accumulate matter and grow larger and larger and larger. There are primordial black holes formed at the beginning of time. There are regular black holes, super massive black holes, and then there are ultra-massive black holes. When a black hole forms from the death of a star and then continues to accumulate things inside of it for billions of years, eventually it becomes a charged black hole. It then generates a powerful outflow of new materials from its center. New stars and planets are then formed from this material.

Here are a couple of parallels between black holes and chakras:

1st. The human body revolves many processes - both physiological and emotional - around the seven chakra centers. In outer space, entire galaxies revolve around black holes.

2nd. The sun can be linked to the cosmic energy that is transformed into human life through the miracle of chakra centers. When the sun dies, it undergoes transformation and becomes a black hole.

Cosmic energy also goes through a death of a certain kind. It gives up its cosmic perspective for an individualized perspective. Because the nature of the black hole is fundamentally different from everything surrounding it, it informs everything surrounding it. Once the star becomes a black hole, it is as if it transforms into another dimension of existence that is operating under different laws than the matter that exists outside of it. It is so incredibly powerful that it affects everything around it and yet no one or nothing can see inside of it to truly understand its power. This is like a chakra center because chakra centers also inform and direct the actions of the physical body and of the mind.

Yet chakras exist in a different dimensional reality other than that which the physical body does. It is said that it takes twice the amount of energy required to run the physical body in order to awaken the first chakra. Then it takes twice that amount to awaken the second and so on and so forth all the way up to the seventh chakra, 128 times the amount of energy it takes to awaken the first chakra.

The difference between black holes and the chakras is that the size is inversely proportional. Chakras exist within the subtle body structure of "Sushumna Nadi." This is the channel of energy that the Kundalini energy travels upward through once it is awakening. It is said to be one thousandth the width of a strand of hair and the chakras exist inside of that one thousandth width of a strand of hair, yet they contain within them power and energy greater than that of a thousand atomic bombs.

When black holes finally emit energy and new stars are formed, we can relate this to the involutionary process of awakening our chakra system and reconnecting to the energy of the sun. Involutionary, not evolutionary, because we are in the process of returning back to our source of becoming one, not many. In this analogy, the sun is like the energy of soul and spirit. The sun means solar, a correlation and derivative of the word soul, hence the word solar plex or the third chakra in which, the associated color is gold. It preceded the black hole but became it when it transformed into the physical body.

When we transform the energy of the physical body back into spirit, our soul generates enough energy to create another sun. In order to get back to the energy of spirit, a great transformation and energy charge has to occur within the chakra system and the body surrounding it. It takes 128 times the energy used to run the physical body to awaken the seventh chakra, or crown chakra. The energy that awakens the chakra system is fundamentally different from the energy that we use on a daily basis to run the physical body. Fundamentally different energy is where the esoteric practices and meditation and yoga come in. It is stillness. Meditation. The greatest athlete to ever live, three-time world heavyweight boxing champion, Muhamed Ali once stated and I quote, " I couldn't be still until I couldn't be still." This was referencing his lengthy battle with Parkinsons disease.

But I took it as a much deeper meaning than that. He learned that there was much more to life than just our primitive nature and that to get to our higher intelligence and nature, we have to just be still, observe and most importantly, listen. Listen to everything within us and around us and connect to the organic and vibrate on the original and higher frequency. So much of the mind is oriented around movement. Movement is a part of matter. Stillness is one of the most difficult goals to achieve on this planet.

Though the Kundalini energy is lying dormant at the base of the spine, there is a fraction of this energy running constantly throughout the body, supporting all of our life processes; and it is made available to us in many ways. If we start engaging in practices that are going to improve the regular physiological and emotional processes that the chakras are influencing, then we can free up an incredible amount of energy that is already here but hidden.

If you still believe that the chakra system is more skepticism than realism, here is proof that they are a real thing and affect our reality in so many ways. I want to introduce you to an article written in 2007 that will pretty much guarantee that this is real and that achieving such feats as transitioning without physically dying seem possible.

CHAKRAS, GALAXIES, AND BLACK HOLES

By Jay Chang, April 11, 2007

S cientific researchers at Jiao Tong University in Shanghai, using sophisticated scientific equipment, have shown that subtle energy has the properties of an electromagnetic current when flowing through acupuncture meridians but takes on the properties of coherent particle streams, similar to laser light when projected out from the body through the hands of master Qigong healers who cure diseases by beaming their energy into the patient's body. There are important chakras on the palms of the hands. To understand how we can beam energy (which is manifested as coherent light) from chakras, some understanding of the structure and dynamics of chakras would be useful.

How do Chakras Form?

Barbara Brennan, former NASA engineer and now world-renowned energy healer, describes chakras as "swirling cone-shaped vortexes in the human energy field." From the perspective of plasma metaphysics, chakras (or "wheels" in Sanskrit) can be considered to be composed of two components: one, a magnetized node, and two, a rotating cone structure or vortex that forms in the low-density magnetic plasma that subtle bodies are composed of.

In laboratory experiments, it has recently been realized that a localized source at a fixed frequency excites a cone of radiation in a plasma crystal. The apex of the cone will be pointed towards the source and the angle of the cone is determined by its spin frequency. Excitations from fast-moving particles in a plane below or next to a single-layered plasma crystal give rise to these cones. According to plasma cosmology, rotating galaxies in space are formed when filamentary currents pinch. This can happen when two currents move towards or cross each other. Dr David Tansely, a radionics specialist, says, "The seven major chakras are formed at points where standing lines of light (or meridians) cross each other 21 times. The 21 minor chakras are located at points where the energy strands cross 14 times." Based on these theories, we can infer how chakras develop in subtle bodies (composed of magnetic plasma or 'magma').

When meridians cross in our subtle bodies, they pinch each other, forming "knots" and collapse as compressed nodes of intense magnetic fields that pulsate at fixed frequencies. Super particles and objects are attracted to the magnetized nodes and are sucked into the subtle bodies at extremely high speeds using helical paths. This dynamical behavior of the incoming particles and the pulsations of the node excite cone structures on the surface of the body. The plasma of charged particles (known popularly in the metaphysical literature as "qi", "prana" or "kundalini"), from the ionized environment, spirals into the nodes, swirling the magnetic plasma on the surface of the compact subtle body. It is then absorbed into the chakra and its energy is then transferred to various parts of the subtle body through the network of meridians (or filamentary currents) within the body.

Structure of Chakras

According to scientific researchers, a complicated elastic double vortex structure emanates from the excited region in a plasma crystal. Each region splits into an outgoing and inward-going vortex. The wavefronts are circular near the source. This resembles how experimental metaphysicists, such as Charles Leadbeater and Brennan, have described and illustrated the spinal chakras - which come in pairs and have circular wavefronts. A tube or channel connects the outward-facing chakra at the front of the body to the chakra behind the body - which faces in the opposite direction.

According to scientific researchers, the cones in plasma crystals possess an interesting multiple structure of nested cones. Nested cones within chakras in our magnetic plasma bodies have been observed by Brennan. According to Brennan, chakras appear "to be nested within each other like nesting glasses. Each chakra on each higher layer extends out farther in the auric field (to the edge of each auric layer) and is slightly broader than the one below it". Each vortex metabolizes an energy that resonates with its particular spin frequency.

Alignment of Chakras

It is interesting to note that the cone structures of chakras are positioned at different angles in illustrations in metaphysical literature. As noted earlier, the angle correlates with the frequency of the radiation source. It is well-known in metaphysics that not only are the spinal chakras positioned at different angles but that each chakra spins at a different frequency. The axis of each cone is aligned with the magnetic field generated by the node so that the apex of the cone of the chakra, which faces the central channels in the subtle body, has a different magnetic polarity from the base of the cone, which faces the environment. If we look at the central channel in the subtle body, the nodes would be distributed along the knots in the central channels at discrete intervals. This agrees well with metaphysical observations (and is consistent with the behavior of magnetic plasma, as noted in studies of plasma crystals). According to Brennan, "Their tips point into the main vertical power current and their open ends extend to the edge of each layer of the field they are located in."

Absorption and Emission of Energy from Chakras

According to Brennan, each swirling vortex of energy appears to suck or entrain energy from the universal energy field. Chakras connect to the nodes of meridians which are areas of intense magnetic fields. They are therefore able to attract high-energy charged super particles and objects. The particles, after absorption, course through the meridians to distribute energy to various parts of the body - similar to what happens in the heart-lung and circulatory systems in the physical-biomolecular body in terms of distributing oxygen to the cells in the body. When particles in subtle bodies are energized, they begin to respond to their environments. Leadbeater explains that one of the functions of chakras is to calibrate (or entrain) the frequencies of particles in order for them to be responsive to particular frequencies of radiation in the environment. Brennan also observes that the direction in which a chakra spins is important. When the chakra is spinning clockwise it is absorbing energy. When spinning anticlockwise - the flow of energy is in the reversed direction. In other words, it is emitting energy rather than absorbing it.

Focused Beams of Light from Rotating Galaxies

According to scientific researchers, an ordered magnetic field plays an essential role in jet formation from a rotating accretion disk in an ionized environment. The process of forming jets (or focused beams of light) is thought to depend on how magnetic fields behave when they are swirled around by an accretion disk. Jets occur in cosmic plasma. As far back as 1918, astronomer H D Curtis noticed a jet from the center of the galaxy M87, describing it as a "curious straight ray" emanating from the galaxy. Taking the form of a huge flashlight beam in space, a jet of electrons and protons traveling at near the speed of light can be seen in NASA's image of the galaxy. The jet is a highly collimated plasma beam (i.e., like coherent laser light). Energetic astrophysical jets, with velocities approaching the speed of light, are seen on a variety of scales emerging from active galactic nuclei and young stars. It is thought that they result from the dynamics of accretion disks rotating around a large mass. The energy radiates from charged particles that are moving in a curved orbit (typically around a magnetic field aligned with the jet).

Focused Beams of Light from Rotating Chakras

The chakra is a rotating accretion disk on a relatively large compact subtle body. We also know (from the above discussion) that the nodes of chakras are locations of intense magnetic fields and charged particles move in helical or spiral paths around this field. Magnetic fields in plasma move with it. The effect of the movement of the particles, plunging into the subtle body at high speeds, is to effectively swirl the intense magnetic field around the axis of the cone of the chakra. This causes the magnetic fields to twist, rise, and eject out as a jet of collimated light. The acceleration mechanism for most jets is magneto hydrodynamic. (Magneto-hydrodynamics provides a general framework to study the activities of magnetic plasma.) The jet being issued will be parallel to the spin axis of the chakra.

Jets or directed beams of light have been seen in photographs taken during events where subtle energetic practices take place (for example: Reiki, Qigong and Christian "Praise and Worship"). There are also Hindu, Taoist, Buddhist and Christian images showing jets of light issuing out from the palms of saints or deities. There are important chakras (and acupoints) on the palms of the hands. The frequency and spin rate of the chakra would have a direct effect in determining the energy and coherence of the beam. One of the seers of the Fatima apparitions of "Mary", "Lucia", revealed that during one of the apparitions, "Mary" opened her hands and "rays of light" issued from them.

This may be done simply by reversing the normal direction of the chakra spin (so that energy is emitted rather than absorbed) and increasing the rotational speed of the chakra in the palm (by mentally focusing on the specific chakra or acupoint in the palm of the hand). Jets may also be issued from other chakras or acupoints - for example from the heart chakra. For example, in the Bible when 'Jesus' appeared to Saint Faustina, two beams of light issued from his heart - one beam was blue and the other was red. Interestingly, jet formations in cosmic objects such as galaxies also show two beams of light - one blue and the other red!

Black Holes and Chakras

According to scientists, black holes also issue jets. In fact, the galaxy M87 (cited above) which issues jets, is suspected to harbor a black hole in its nucleus. (The black hole is then analogous to the node and the galaxy to the cone structure of the chakra.) This is surprising because, as far as we know, the strong gravitational fields of black holes absorb energy - letting nothing escape. (Small black holes, though, give out Hawking radiation.) If we use the same explanation as we did for chakras, this may be because of the direction of the spin of the accretion disks around black holes. Does this mean that if the direction of the spin of the accretion disk of a rotating ("Kerr") black hole is reversed it will start ejecting energy instead of absorbing it? Black holes with highly energetic jets spin the fastest, according to scientists.

If we further apply what we have learned about the structure of chakras to black holes, we expect black holes to come in pairs. Each black hole would then be connected by a tube (popularly called a " wormhole") which connects to another black hole in another part of our universe. This wormhole may be long or very short - so that there is a double vortex structure (like in chakras) connected by a short tube - giving rise to jets that eject in opposite directions from astrophysical objects. Astrophysical jets that emanate from opposite directions of astrophysical objects have been seen. We would also expect black holes to reside within all galaxies as they are simply entry points into the network or web of "meridians" (in this case filamentary currents) that transfer energy from one point to another, throughout the universe.

To carry the analogy with chakras further, this would imply that black holes and galaxies are formations in an invisible subtle body - the subtle body of our universe. This also suggests that this subtle body is composed of (dark) magnetic plasma. We are living inside the subtle body of this universe - on a planet that is sitting on the edge of one of its chakras - a chakra we call the Milky Way.

All of these things that I have discussed - melanin, the seven chakras, and the pineal gland - are our God-given powers and abilities. We should use these to our advantage when faced with hatred and death from our oppressors. These are weapons of omnipotence and something to fight with. These "weapons" as I call them, can stand against the armies of the world.

I reflect back on the scripture; "No weapons formed against me shall prosper." The kingdom is ours; the power is ours and ultimately in the end the glory is ours. So, as I continue in my 43 years, I'm wondering, how can we get back to this infinite power? Ultimately, understanding our melanin as it relates to the universe, to the chakras, and to the pineal gland... that's spiritual. Economically, in America, 1.3 trillion dollars can be credited to the Black dollar, yet not even about 3% of this amount circulates back into the Black community.

This is why it is so important to spend our money supporting each other and other Black-owned businesses. There is Heaven in winning, and hell in not trying. One way to keep a race of people in an inferior state is to keep that race depending on their oppressors. By spending money with Black-owned businesses and corporations like Black-owned banks, restaurants, real estate, educational, and religious institutions (that teach the rebirth of Black consciousness and not this watered-down, brainwashing of and from the scriptures inside Christian churches and Islamic mosques), we can rebound in a powerful way, because we depend on ourselves, each other.

We should educate our people in what we know and not what we speculate. Like, I stated earlier, we should have Black wall streets all over the nation. Black churches should be community driven, and economically relevant, teaching the truth about the science and spirituality of the African religious system. We should invest our wealth in the hands of those who understand first-hand how hard it is for us and the struggles we carry as a race of people. Who better to invest in, than each other, ourselves?

Third Eye Publishing

PART III

My Life Outside of The Heavens, Inside the Earth, with Mahogany

Third Eye Publishing

]

FOUR BEAUTIFUL DAUGHTERS: ZHARIA, TIMILLE, AUTUMN, AND NADIA

Most of what makes me who I am is because of the special woman who has been here in my life through all of this self-destruction and self-reconstruction of what is Timothy V. Lane. Her name is Mahogany. I have never met someone who can tolerate so much, but still produce so much love and compassion. As strong as she is beautiful, she will give her all so that her children and family can have it all. She is truly the Earth, the world to me. Though I am instinctively drawn and possessed by the Heavens, I tend to run into Mahogany's presence when searching for them.

She is the gateway into the heart and soul of the Heavens. Mahogany Byrd. An Angel who takes flight and soars up into the innermost part and being of the Heavens. She is loyal and humble, the epitome of everything that the Heavens want to be. She is free to the outside universe but chooses to stay within the comfort and protection of my love for her, knowing that there is no other love greater. And she deserves everything positive that she has coming to her. She has given me four beautiful daughters, Zharia, Timille, Autumn, and Nadia.

Everything that I am and aim to be, I owe to them. To be a better husband, a better man, and most importantly, a better father. Living with someone who suffers from mental illness can weigh on the hearts and minds of those who love them most, which is why I have decided to include them in this book and let them vent about what they deal with living with a schizophrenic. Some of the things I have done to them are a little harsh or maybe even unforgivable. But still, I am just trying my best to deal the cards I was dealt in life.

Even with that, I love my family religiously. I would not do anything to intentionally hurt them. I have said hurtful, evil things out of anger, but I love them so much. I just really want them (my kids) to do better and go further than me. Look, I make no excuses for the things that I have done to hurt my family and a few close friends. But it's like I am screaming out to Heaven and Earth from my innermost core. Hoping to reach their innermost core. It's one thing to lust after women, but it is a completely different ball game when we are talking about being in love with one's soul. Life is about balance and maintaining the balance of soul and flesh, good and evil, Heaven and Earth, positive and negative.

The weight of this world is heavy, and it is a tremendous struggle to rise and stand with the weight I am carrying on my shoulders. I don't know where I am getting my strength now. My legs are buckling, but I continue to lift, because Heaven and Earth depend on me to lift them. They depend on me to maintain the balance in nature as well as in the cosmos. The fact that I am still here dealing with the pressure is a testament and proof that God is here, right here in the here and now, waiting for the return and rebirth of Black consciousness and the re-establishment of the Black family back to prominence and royalty on this planet. So, I will start with re-establishing my own family, building back, and reinstating their confidence in me. I want to give them a chance to tell their side of the story. I want them to let the world know what it is like living with a schizophrenic.

LIVING WITH
A SCHIZOPHRENIC

This is my family's perspective on what it's like living with someone who suffers with mental illness:

Living with a person who deals with Schizophrenia can be a very harrowing experience. It can be tumultuous. It can be draining. The best way I can describe it is like the feeling of sitting through a bad storm. You know that slightly frightening moment when you can see the lightning in the sky, but haven't heard a roaring clap of thunder yet? You know it's going to happen; you just don't know when. And you know it's going to be loud; you just don't know how loud it's actually going to be. Loud enough to shake your house, loud enough to wake you up from your sleep. Loud enough that you actually feel your heart skip a beat. That's what it feels like. You know something might happen at any second of the day, you just don't know to what degree.

There are levels to it. It's noisy 90% of the time. Noisy like the wind from that bad storm that we were talking about earlier. Noisy like rain hitting your roof, insistent and consistent in a way. Like the rain not only wants to be heard, but it *needs* to be. The noise can be manageable. But nothing is as scary as when they have their bouts of paranoia. Or when they get into a self-deprecating mood. It overtakes not only the person with the illness but everyone around them too. That's when that heavy rain turns to flooding. When it turns into a tidal wave. It turns into something you can see coming, but you, yourself, can't stop it. And when it all hits you, it hurts. But you have to remind yourself that the water didn't mean to hurt you, that's just what it does. It's in nature, so can you really be upset with it? You learn how to not take it personally; the water doesn't decide where it lands. Gravity does.

The ill don't always decide how they react, the disease does that for them sometimes. It makes you wonder. That's another feeling you have to deal with… confliction, that is. "He's yelling at me, is this him or the illness?" "He's being very rude today, is this him or the illness?" Those are questions you have to ask yourself. It takes a long time to separate the person from the thoughts that plague their mind. "Am I allowed to react? Am I allowed to be mad right now?" More questions you will ask yourself. And if you as a person with a healthy mind are wondering these things, you can only imagine what the brain of the unhealthy is thinking at the moment.

Don't think too hard about that. Their brain is a cacophony of things. It's colorful like a wall of graffiti or like a stained-glass window. Sometimes you get those calm moments, where everything is good. They're laughing, they're joking around. And you hope it stays that way. You hope the sun stays out and dries up all the water that's on the pavement. You hope the brightness washes over you as hard as the tidal wave did. For when the sun is out, and the light is bright, everything is peaceful. Birds are singing and kids are laughing like you're living inside a cheesy movie. Like you've finally reached the eye of the storm where everything stops for a moment, and you feel safe and content. And when they're in the eye with you, they teach you things. They share things with you. Whether that be deep, dark secrets, or something as simple as their favorite comic book character. They cook the family dinner, or they play video games with you. They recite scripture to you, or they sit and watch a movie and ask 100 questions. You get annoyed because you are trying to watch, but you answer anyway, because it has finally stopped raining, and you feel better than you did yesterday. When they're happy, it makes you happy, it makes everyone happy really because it feels normal. It feels much better than constantly fearing that loud clap of thunder you've been waiting to hear these past few minutes. It's quiet and when it rains so often, you need it to be.

—-From, the family.
Written by my oldest daughter, Zharia

Life is about change and transition. I believe that we are put here on this planet to strive for perfection. How can we be perfect in our craft if we don't evolve and change a few things about the way to approach certain obstacles? So, in my mind, I can't stop until my and my family's souls turn into solid gold. That is the true wealth. Knowledge and wisdom become power, the crowning moment of perfection.

Knowing the ins and outs of who we are as a people who derived from tremendous wealth is a way back to that tremendous wealth. The only way to get that back is by knowing who you are, or who you were before you became brainwashed by the heavy European influence. So, I would like to start with the very thing that made us so hated in the first place… Our skin pigment.

The study of melanin is the study of alchemy. It is the process of learning how to transform the particles or metals in the human body as well as the universe (both one in the same) into pure gold, which shines brighter than the sun.

Third Eye Publishing

PART IV

Blessings in Blackness

Third Eye Publishing

MELANIN MAGIC:
NADIA

W hen discussing melanin, we cannot go fully in-depth without discussing the pineal gland and melatonin. The pineal gland is an organ that is found in the center of the brain. This gland, also referred to as the inner or third eye, is approximately the size of a single kernel of corn.

Ancestrally it was well known that the pineal gland, or third eye, was the seat of the soul, and when properly activated, it would allow us to then move from our lower nature to our higher intelligence and selves. Activation of the pineal gland was believed to allow us to meet God face to face. This process is even referred to in the Bible. Genesis 32:30-31 reads: "And Jacob called the name of the place Pineal, for I have seen God face to face and my life is preserved. And as he passed over Pineal, the sun rose upon him." That is just one of some 69 references in the Bible. The pineal gland is the first gland developed in your body and appears in homo-sapiens a mere three weeks after conception. There are five things that the pineal gland is responsible for.

1. Inner eye- sensing light and darkness

2. The biological clock tells our bodies when to do its functions.

3. Pacemaker- sets the pace or rhythm for the body.

4. Compass- helps us orient ourselves.

5. Production and secretion of two biologically key harmonies: The pineal gland is responsible for producing and secreting the hormones serotonin and melatonin. Serotonin is secreted during the daylight hours. Melatonin is secreted in the nighttime hours. These hormones work inversely.

6. The pineal gland is influenced by several things that allow it to function properly.

Light, more specifically natural sunlight

Temperature

Food, particularly green raw vegetables because of the chlorophyll, which is plant melanin.

Sleep is important for the production of melatonin. Science has shown a direct correlation between night and the secretion of melatonin. It reaches its max at midnight.

It is important to note that melatonin is to be produced and secreted at night while you are sleeping. Therefore, a decrease in melatonin or too much melatonin production during daylight can cause depression. It has several distinct functions. It boosts memory, intensifies REM or dream sleep, organizes our system biologically, mentally, and spiritually, slows aging, strengthens the immune system, puts us in a pleasant mood, and resets our biological clock, which helps us adapt to new environments/time zones.

Melatonin creates melanin. Melanin is a chemical substance that gets secreted in the blood. It is primarily responsible for the pigmentation of our skin, but also serves in other capacities.

The function of melanin is to serve as a natural sunscreen. It protects humans from UV rays from the sun, and protects against skin cancer, Parkinson's disease, and radiation. Scientific research has also shown that melanin has several life sustained benefits:

1. It is believed to counterattack stress.

2. Minimize jet lag.

3. regulate biological rhythms.

4. And may even protect against cancer and heart disease.

Melanin is not produced by accident or by chance, the production of melanin requires certain nutrients - particularly amino acids. A nutrient deficiency will cause the melanin to be recessive or virtually inactive, manifesting in very light, or pale skin pigmentation, as well as light hair and light-colored eyes. If the proper nutrients are in place, the melanin will manifest in black/dark brown skin, dark hair, and dark eyes. Therefore, depigmentation is a direct correlation to the genetic inability to produce a sufficient amount of melanin. Scientifically, there are six classifications of melanin:

> **Types 1/2/3** are referred to as having pheo-melanin 1 are those that are "Caucasian," Euros that are often Irish, Welsh, and Scottish.

> **Type 4** are lightly tanned; Japanese, Chinese, Italians, Greek, and Spanish, and some Indians fall into this type.

> **Type 5** ranges from brown skin to very dark Black skin. These are Mexicans, Malaysians, Puerto Ricans, and many South American inhabitants.

> **Type 6** true or EU melanin is found in this type: Egyptian, Ethiopian, Nigerians, African Americans, Australian Aborigines all make type 6. These people are as close to Gods and Goddesses or Superheroes as you are going to get. Because of the greater melanin pigment, they are deeply connected and deeper rooted to the mysteries of the universe and the cosmos.

As I stated earlier, the study of melanin is also the study of alchemy. It is the study of turning particles and metals in the body as well as the universe into pure gold. Gold is the greatest conductor of energy and electricity. Once the chakras are aligned and rotating at the proper rate and activated, one will begin to experience "Siddhis" and illuminate. Pure light will be permeated throughout every part of our being and we will be able to tap into superhuman strength and superhuman intelligence. We will be able to see a wider, more advanced view of the astrological plane as opposed to what we can experience in this Earthly realm. We become one with electromagnetic fields and can cross over into any celestial, terrestrial and astral plane. These planes are cerebral but are also connected to the cosmos. It is believed that an astral plane houses the angels of Heaven, and other non-terrestrial beings and the souls of the past who once dwelled on the Earth, all of whom make up the 12 constellations or the sky as we observe it.

Electricity generated from the ground when we step onto the soil is absorbed throughout our being and also generated from the Earth's electromagnetic field and other electromagnetic fields across other astrological planes. These electromagnetic charges transform us into pure light, we become solar, electric beings with electromagnetic energy and electricity being absorbed by our crystallized (Referring to the word Christos or Christ because of the crystallization of stars) Melanin and then emitted throughout every part of our body; beacons of golden light shining through. This supernatural feat is known as "the anointing" or the state of the immaculant and divine powers.

When the Pineal gland or the third eye is opened and activated, we see into other dimensions more than just these 3 dimensions in which we experience on this side of life. Our crown or 7th chakra is activated, and we become the sun, bright golden light. When this happens, we become supernatural; pure light, there will be no need for the stars, sun, or moon for this is the light and energy of the world and of the universe.

It is the glory of God and of the Messiah (Revelations 21:23). It is the brilliance of the higher intelligence. It burns with great and bright wisdom like candles in a dark room and is the lamp of life and existence. It beams through him and his people with a golden light shining brighter than any star. It is the shine of all knowing knowledge, power, brilliance, and wisdom. In the scriptures, it says that there will be no more sickness, no more pain, and no more death. Evidently, there will be knowledge of cures, we will know how to heal sickness and pain. Hueman beings will be impervious to disease.

It goes along to say that God will wipe away all tears, and he will be their God and they will be his people, and there will be no more death. This will happen to an individual first, and then it will be spread out to anyone who believes his theology and the evidence to back it up with the science. There is a story in the New Testament that talks about how Jesus and his disciples were in a boat traveling across the sea headed to a certain destination. The disciples noticed that Jesus was not on the boat when a storm arose. They became fearful that they were not going to arrive at their destination. One of the disciples looked out on the water and saw Jesus walking on the water. Then he stepped out on the water in faith because his Messiah told him too and he began to walk. Then he began to doubt and started to sink. It was at this time Jesus grabbed his hand and walked him toward the boat. Afraid that they wouldn't reach their destination in time, and still hundreds of miles away from shore, the disciples cried out to Jesus and when he approached and boarded the boat, immediately they arrived at their destination.

This to me is a metaphor and symbolism, a story describing the power of the anointing and the effect that it and the Messiah will have on his people once they encounter him. They mentally, spiritually, and physically will immediately arrive at their destination; on his train of thought, intelligence, power, wisdom, and frequency, and they will be transformed and changed forever. A new being, a new creature they will become.

Once people witness, they will follow. He himself is a black hole, a dead star that will consume and absorb any entity, mind, body, and soul. Evidently, this will be some sort of universal scientific breakthrough as we will have evolved as a species into supernatural, highly intelligent super hueman beings understanding our mind and bodies and how they relate to the nature of the universe.

It is coming 360 degrees back into our own knowledge, conscious and being, back to the original source vibrating on a higher frequency, our original frequency. We will see everything, feel everything, and hear everything. Our senses will be so heightened and sensitive we will be in tune and one with everything within and around us. It is THE GREAT AWAKENING, the rebirth of black consciousness when Black people wake from their slumber and spiritual death and realize who they are, and that power and wealth is theirs. This is beginning to happen now.

This is a scientific explanation of the spiritual golden city, the Kingdom of Heaven as it is described in the Bible. Not to be focused on as a physical place, per say, but more so of a state of mind and being, Sapio. Once this feat is achieved by him, his people will achieve the same feat and in the same way. He and his people (Israel) are one and are very capable of unlocking the mysteries of death and the universe. This is the science of transitioning without physically dying. This is the mystery and the magic of melanin, and why the government, (white) Amerikkka, is spending over $500,000,000 a year on melanin research.

Comprehending this typography is important in order to understand one essential characteristic of melanin. Melanin in its purest form is jet black. It is the deepest black because of its ability to absorb and store energy. The reason melanin in its purest form shows up black is because the chemical structure will not allow any type of energy to escape. The more energy that is absorbed the darker the melanin and therefore the darker the pigmentation. Type 5 and 6 are able to absorb the most energy. Types 1 and 3 are melanin recessive and therefore instead of absorbing energy they reflect it; this is particularly evident with light energy because when light energy is reflected it shows up white. The difference between pheo melanin and eumelanin can be distinguished scientifically by the amount of sulfur present in the melanin. Eumelanin was found to have 0-1% sulfuric presence. And pheo-melanin 1 was found to have 9-12% sulfuric concentration.

So, while whites do have a pineal gland, their gland is calcified and does not produce melanin in abundance. It is believed that melanin responds to and absorbs light energy, sound energy (specifically through music) and electrical energy and uses the absorbed energy to disperse to parts of the body like a nutrient. Creating a symbiotic relationship, melanin is essentially involved in the mental and physical aspects of every part of the body in a melanin-dominated (type 5 and 6) person. Melanin is also known to be necessary for proper receptivity to energy in the external environment. Everything in nature emits some kind of energy. Melanin keeps types 5 and 6 tuned with the great ability to be aware and intuitive regarding their surrounding environment. Again, it is especially important that we, eumelanated people, keep our pineal gland activated so that it can act in a manner that it was designed to produce melanin and melatonin. Again, how do we activate our pineal gland?

1. Sunlight- it is very important for eumelanated people to spend time in natural light.

2. Chlorophyll- in the form of green vegetables, raw is best.

3. Sleep- before midnight as we see a significant spike in melanin at that time.

4. Water- another purifier for the body, it helps release toxins.

5. Good music and other strong vibratory frequencies- this is particularly important for the pineal gland.

The universe is made of melanin. The pineal gland inside of the brain produces melanin. This is my theory. We live inside a living, thinking entity, and that living, thinking entity is entrapped and living inside of us. An entity that I think is two, is made one by the marriage of consciousness and material, or energy and matter, the stars and space. It is the yin and the yang, man and woman. I think this is why marriage is recognized by God as the union between man and woman. It, to me, is the only logical explanation. Yes, there is one God, but yet again there are more than one (man and woman, father and mother, or God and a Goddess) the combination constitutes the marriage, and we, as beings, created in their image are the direct result of that combination, union, and marriage.

I also believe that this is why the commandment, "Honor thy Mother and thy Father, so that thy days will be long on this earth," is one of the first given. It is for the continued existence of the hueman race on planet Earth. This is a natural thing and should be taught as such in the schools and churches. Homosexuality runs rampant throughout this country. Someone once said to me, "If God is going to let

America continue to be what it is today, then he owes Sodom and Gamora an apology." I really couldn't disagree with that statement. It is the truth. Amerikkka has become the one thing that it escaped from, an oppressor. Now oppressing the minds of the youth, programming them to believe that it is okay to live that lifestyle. Amerikkka has made homosexuality mainstream.

Leviticus 18:22 and 20:13 calls homosexuality an abomination. Roman's 1:26-28 calls homosexuality a vile affection and that it is practiced by the reprobate. If you don't know what a reprobate is, it is an unprincipled person, a person without moral principles. I have always said that homosexuality was driven by lust, more so than love. Homosexuals say that they are born this way, I think that they have deceived themselves.

The reason I say that is because when they say that they are born this way, it is like a slap in the face to God and humanity. That is saying that you don't have a brain to choose who you will serve, God or your own desires. It is a lustful, selfish act and it's not natural and that is what makes it an abomination.

Besides, it is not how life can be created. Creation is life. Life is family, and on that note, I can't help but to revert back to what I consider family. My Heaven, my Earth (Mahogany) now have become my family due to deeply, spiritually rooted connections that will forever link us together.

I have four daughters with Mahogany, but I can't help but believe that on a macro level, the children of the world belong to Heaven and me. To me, the Heavens and Mahogany are one, and I am one with whatever is inside of them connecting them to me.

They say that God is always on time. On the contrary, "Hell is the truth seen too late," as someone once said to me. The realization of who Black people are, as a people, has to be manifested from what is inside of us as a whole. We are souls. That is really what this boils down to, our souls.

All of the knowledge and wisdom that I have I have attained and provided in these two books, I have tried to share with not only Heaven and Earth, but with OUR children as well. It has to come back to me. That energy or the souls, which are the light, belong to me. It made you who you are. You are more than just a "hueman." You are the image of God. God is the family, and that is what is and has been destroyed among so many of us throughout generations, the family.

Getting back to Hell being the truth seen too late, everything in my life seemed to arrive late in life. I was a late developer, not developing until later in high school, which led to me being picked on and bullied a lot.

A dream that I had when I was eight years old was to be the Heavyweight Boxing Champion of the World. This dream went unnoticed by people who could have steered me in that direction until I was eighteen. By then, I had a taste of the street life, and I could not properly dedicate myself to the craft the way that I wanted to, or how I should have. We never had cable when I was growing up and I missed a lot of the big fights and boxing news that would have inspired me to want to be the best and stay away from the alcohol, the women, and the weed.

I felt like this was purposely done to me and something did not want me to have confidence. I put so much energy into the sport that turned out to be wasted on my dreams. This continued until I was eighteen. I had already lost before I could begin. *Did I see the truth too late?* Another instance in which I saw the truth too late was when I first had the memory of Heaven Starr come back to me at the age of nineteen. I had a vision that the girl I was searching for from my past all of this time, was burning in a fire of lust. I couldn't get the vision out of my head, so I wrote a poem about it called "To Fight for a Heaven Starr."

This was at a time when I was a 19-year-old boy searching for a 19-year-old girl. I did not find her until I was twenty-five. She was a virgin when we graduated high school, but I couldn't get to her before the world swallowed her up. So now, I find myself digging deep within myself, hoping to find something powerful enough to bring her out of the depths; Still fighting. *(The poem called "To Fight for a Heaven Starr" is currently in my first book. "Trapped

Inside My Mind: Dimensions and Black and White Poetry from the Perspective of a Schizophrenic.") In this sense, I ask you, is Hell the truth seen too late? Do I even need to mention the other female named Heaven who found me that same year in 1998? At the time, she also had been a virgin at the age of twenty-one.

Now granted, I have mental illness, but I couldn't help but believe that God was toying with me. This was just no coincidence. This, to me, meant something. Whatever it was, and whatever it meant eluded me. For whatever reason, I could not capitalize on, or even process what was happening to me. All of this, while getting turned onto new knowledge and information on the true worth of Black people.

Everything was pointing toward Black people in the universe and the universe being Black people. Back then, in the late 90s. This kind of mindset would have been powerful, leading us into the new millennium, and beyond. But because we failed to look deeper, me, Mahogany, and the Heavens included, prolonged our psychological captivity and enslavement even longer.

What a lot of people don't understand is that everyone wants to be the chosen people of God. The fact of the matter is that the Jews are among the richest people on Earth. True Israel is spread out to the four corners of the Earth and according to the Bible - (Deuteronomy 28 and Leviticus 46) these people are suffering. They are at the bottom of society, suffering from the curses placed upon them by

God for worshiping pagan gods and pagan religions. I got this information in 1999, but no one wanted to believe it or hear it. We know from scripture that when God turns his back on a spiritually dead Israel because they wouldn't "wake up," this realm will be destroyed. So now I ask you, "Did God come right on time, or for Black people, is Hell the truth seen too late?"

I constantly hear the voices screaming at me, saying "It's too late, it's too late," and then I will hear another voice saying to me "Tim, it's okay. You won. Yours is stronger." I still don't exactly know for sure what they mean or what they are trying to get me to believe. *Is it too late for me and Heaven, or too late to save the world? Is it too late to save my people? Or is it too late for those who mistreated us (Black people)?*

When the voices tell me I won, what does that mean? *Did I win the battle against Zeus and the Christians with this talk of an awakening? Did they just finally give in to me because I wouldn't quit fighting to get Heaven and Earth back? Or did I win against the people oppressing our people? Did I win against God, and assure Lucifer a place back into the kingdom? Or did I win against the evil of the world, Satan, who has denied me of my joy, happiness, and confidence over my lifetime?*

It's hard to determine right now. So many traps are set to affect my thought process or thinking pattern. Living with Schizophrenia, I find it hard to trust anything or anyone. Even my own thoughts are questioned. Even though it's tough, I still know one thing for sure, I know that this planet used to belong to Black people. I also know that we as a people are at the bottom of the totem pole in society. I also know that before anyone can see Christ again this world must fall back under the control of Black people. This world began with a Hamitic, king and queen (Adam & Eve). And it must end with the king and queen.

We are headed into the New World Order, where there will be one belief system, one government, one currency, one king, and one queen. This has already been set in motion. It is set up for a being to rise and take the necessary steps to ascend to the throne. The funny thing is this talk was started and enhanced by George H.W. Bush, in the late 80s, but no one knows who this person will be. In the Bible, it is said that this person will be of Israeli descent. That could be any Black person in the Americas, being that true Israel is said to be lost, and spread out to the four corners of the Earth. Suffering from the given curses placed on them.

The number 666 actually refers to the number of the "hueman." Man was created on the sixth day. The sixth element is carbon. Carbon is black or brown and this is what our universe is made of… melanin. Melanin or black is also the hue of the original beings on the planet. 666 is 6 electrons, 6 protons, and 6 neutrons. This is the makeup of the carbon atom, the universe, or in Christianity, our father the Atom, or (Adam). This is why I stated earlier that this world began with Adam and Eve, a Hamitic king and queen, and it will end with a Black king and queen, of course, the word "ham" meaning Black.

So even though this New World Order was put in motion by our own enemies, to directly control the masses (Black people) it is actually set up for a Black person to achieve and become. The Bible says that the first will be the last, and the last will be the first. For me, this has never been more evident than now. I don't claim to be the smartest person in the world, but I can make sense out of things that don't make sense, like this universe. To European scientists, it does not make sense, but to me, it's as simple as a man meets a woman. And in that, there lies the marriage of the stars and matter, and also the creation of life.

As a person who suffers from Schizophrenia, it's not hard for me to take something as complicated as this universe and life, and make it look simple, which is one of the joys of being different. However, I find it extremely difficult to tackle simple everyday tasks and obstacles. That is the curse of the disease. Look, my family has been through hell and back dealing with this. From my parents to my sister, to my cousins, and my immediate family. I have been cruel, and sometimes just downright mean to some of them. I make no excuses, but a lot of what's going on with me may not be entirely in my control. My family members used to say to me that the voices are not them. If that's the case, then, who have I been communicating with? What if it's an entity from another realm or dimension, disguising themselves as my family members? As for my surviving family, most of them have shied away from me. They don't come to visit or invite me anywhere; they don't call me or make time to check on me. Most of my cousins act like they don't give a damn about me. My own mother has turned against me, it seems probably fed up with my constant disrespect.

All that I can say to them is that I'm sorry. I apologize for not being able to remember the Tim that they all once loved and had fun with. That Tim has been murdered by who exists now, which is only me, myself, and I. This Tim is focused on bringing Black people back to prominence on this planet. In the words of one of our heroes, Malcolm, X, "By any means necessary."

I have no feelings inside except a feeling of anxiousness for justice for my slaughtered people. My soul is dark, and in that I find light. My conscience expands and is one with the universe. The way that I think, most would say that I am out of my mind. I would like to say that I think outside of the box. In my last book, I talk about the six sides, which are six directions that we can experience in this life. There is up and there is down. There is a front to back. There is a side to side. This equals six. A box or cube. Which, of course, is the carbonated universe. I guess you can say that I think outside of that box. Though this serves me well with this occupation, for the better part of 25 years or so, I have not been able to hold down a job for more than two years. I was always hypnotized by thoughts of Heaven, thoughts of absolute power, and undeniable knowledge, and unmatched wisdom. Not just for me, but also for my people… people who look and sound like me. The fact that I couldn't keep a job affected me in ways which are hard for me to talk about. My confidence, in many ways, was already shot, took a direct hit, and all of a sudden, I had no motivation. I became depressed and forced to do things out of my character just to support my weed habit. Things I am too ashamed to talk about. Let's just say I hate askin' people for shit. People are constipated. Anyway, I would not reveal these things to you, if I did not care deeply about you or someone you know who suffers from mental illness. Not saying that I have all of the answers, but at least I can point most people (woke or not) in the right direction. Some (woke or not) may not even choose a direction, a path of faith to walk individually for themselves. Some (woke or not) are content to being followers and to follow others (religions).

You have to have a belief in yourself and an understanding of what is happening to you. Someone once told my mother when I was first diagnosed 25 years ago, to save everything that I write. My mother must have known that I was destined to be an author, because she still has to this day, the first book I ever wrote and illustrated 39 years ago. A book on Thunder Cats. I was six years old then. So, if these two books that I have written now become bestsellers, I plan to have that Thundercat book framed and laminated. And this is my will, if I die, all that I make from being an author belongs to my Mahogany, and my four daughters, my niece, my sister, and my mother and father. My Heaven, My Earth, My Family.

PART V

My Poetic World

Third Eye Publishing

(2023)
THIS IS POETIC TELEKINESIS

This is poetic telekinesis; I move souls like planets and stars around these poetic pieces. I am moving people like a planetary alignment, aligning their mind with stardom, freeing them from centuries of psychological solitary confinement. With each piece, the need to educate and inform them increases. As I try to define, the esoteric practices of the soul, flesh and mind, the quest to defeat death never, in my mind, ceases. If I, for whatever reason, seem to find an answer, just remember that if you keep believing you too will discover immortality and then like me, you will become a master. You ask, *what is in the hereafter?* Just think of everything that you as a terrestrial being can physically see with your eyes; that is only 10% of what is actually here. The other 90% is what is imagined by you, and in that there lies the prize. So just think of how close it is, it's near.

What I had to realize was that there was more than what meets the eye, and to transform what is, meant to look past what was, which is what I could see. And move what was beyond my sight. In that movement I gained true power and might. In that moment, I learned my true identity. In that might, I never meant to knock heaven down into pieces, with Sacred Eternal Xtascy. My true insight was to move what was behind her gates and within her walls. The spirits within were moving to my words and word. And that word was that I would never be leaving. So that is what I am believing. That I am immortal, the one that paid the cost, operating on our original frequency. I know that power and peace is stillness, but I am moving what is behind the scenes frequently. Remembering how I was able to achieve the ability, I share what I have learned and hope in all directions it reaches; The masses of the people and reign stability, I really believe this, we need this, this is our resiliency, this is spiritual, lyrical, poetic telekinesis.

(2018)
TO THE YOUNG BLACK MALE:
OUR YOUNG BLACK UNIVERSE

Our young black universe, do you know where you are? Not to say that you don't, but if you don't, look within, and home won't be far. The Atom or Adam, energy of all energies, frequency of all frequencies which was conceived by your wife, the sky at night, your Eve. This is why you believe in thee.

Love is why she gave and saved your life, the life that she gave you, you beheld the beauty. You remembered what saved you when she loved you truly. She is the space, you are the star, remember what brought you to grace, and remember what brought you this far. You are the seed, she will carry you in her womb, protected and reflected just as the sun, earth, and moon.

Our Young Black Universe, tell me, do you know of your worth? Your skin is as valuable as oil because you are the earth. Your soul is sought out by races of every nation and creed because it is as valuable as gold to a spiritually poverty-stricken world that is desperately in need. But be careful of those who are driven by greed, remember to dispatch your wealth honorably to those who deserve it. Turn away those who have evil intentions or do evil deeds.

Our Young Black Universe, do you remember our cycling times, electrons and protons revolving around neutrons, and the nucleus of the atom. Planets and moons revolve around our sun, you are the future, and something that we cannot fathom as you continue to revolve around our minds. You are something for everyone.

Our young black universe, remember why you are here. The world is yours, so seize it, with the strength of the lord. To control, command, and have no fear. Fear no man, demon, or beast, for you are the angel of the lord. The life inside of you has called you into existence, to be at peace, so stabilize, grow infinite and wise. And, our lives will be your reward, and in that, your life will never cease.

True power is only realized and defined in the form of the absolute, well we have absolute power, when we lean toward the mind and the meditation of the creation of you. Truth, I say, will always recognize truth. That is the original atom or that frequency saying to you, I'm here, I've always been here. That is the you in me, and the me in you too."

So, continue to listen to the earth, those voices that revolve around the sun which is your mind; they will keep you in tune with reality, and your worth. They will keep you making the right choices; ultimately, keeping you and the heavens intertwined for everyone.

Young black universe, you are my seed, your mother's nature has watered you with the cosmic waters of existence until your mind grew infinite. Now, we hope to have a place in your kingdom, so please remember your mother and me. For it was our love in which how you came to be, and it will be love that will one day grant us eternity.

Forgive us all for the ignorance we showcase when placed in your vast intelligence we forget how amazing grace is when we are all concerned with ourselves and how we live as if the world is irrelevant. The eloquence and the words in which you spoke and molded life's form into her being is evident in our role in nature's play and in which we function as if life is only as real as what we are believing.

Still receiving the best that life has to offer, it is you, young black universe who should receive this knowledge of who we are so we can prosper, and if for any man-made reason there should be any inward treason know that no matter what, they cannot destroy you, or put an end to your season. What is within us is what we should all be believing for that is life, something we can give to the subjects who cannot live; we breathe in them, and then they begin breathing.

Young black universe, never be ashamed of your darkness, your dreams and possibilities burn like an inferno. The melanin in your skin makes the impossible possible. These words will be the event that sparked it. Others not used to you will fear you because you are dark, they will not understand why you wear your nappy hair the way you do, or why you are the heir to infinite wealth. The kingdom which is you. Your thoughts run long, just as Africa's Nile River irrigating the cosmos, the land around it, as you become the life-giver. Son, you are the sun and now I am yours. Shed light on those who have none, to them you are lord. Never let doubt make you feel as if you cannot achieve, for the only thing to doubt is the fact that they cannot defeat you. Remember that for the micro-ones who look up to you and believe.

Our young black universe, my soul is yours. I am living, and working, so your creation can soar, however it be or whatever I have to travel through. I will do so with pride, so I can see the best of you, your purpose here is to unite and bring balance to the creation. Stand up for those who cannot fight for justice and do so without hesitation.

Young black universe, we are no richer than the poorest man and no poorer than the richest. Remember that young black universe and we can feed all the people in the promised land, for peace is the reason you are here. You are energy and that energy is to be used to fight for that only. No matter what you have to endure, as a man thinketh he is, so think like a messiah and that's how much higher we all can live.

It is your power and that is what we all have to give. To redeem you with this vote of confidence so you can replenish us and make us pure with the love you created us with. Trusting that we will all come through for you, so you can come through for us, and bring into existence a world of love, with materials and enough wealth to heal starvation, bringing peace in a new world built on trust.

Young black universe, give praise to your melanin. For your pigment is vast and is the reason men search for ultimate truths; to bring knowledge to their brethren the intriguement of past creations and how we are made better as a man with hue. So be not ashamed of your darkness for it is in that, that we discover new jewels, gems, and fuel. Fuel for the galactic minds to chastise and test the hearts of mortal men, only then do we realize who the real heroes of the universe are and what we are really up against.

Let not your heart be troubled by the suffering of the very people who created you; with you, a new day is dawning, and the light is starting to shine through. Your ancestors have prayed hard for your deliverance. Now stand on this, you are more than man; you are the Amen, the original source, the atom or Adham, whose name means black blood or dark red earth.

You are a God to this creation, so believe so and take back the Earth. You have to for all it is worth because it is the only known life in this universe. Until I see another, I will believe that we are the only ones who can reach everyone in one thought simply because we are number one.

We are the blueprint or foundation that each nation is built on. So be proud of who you are and let your aura be loud, so loud that they recognize it and know that you are king. Our young black universe, you are everyone's dream. As I continue to bring to you this revelation of who I am inside of you and who you are inside of me, I must believe that we are all one because that is the only way for us to have peace, at least that is the way it seems. It seems as if they want to destroy you because you are the very source of the power. They hate you because you are knowledge and wisdom beyond what they can conceive. They do heinous things to try to annoy you to the point where you make a mistake and then feed off of your misery, and then they have rain to shower.

Beware, young black universe, for you have much to devour. The hour has come for you to feed on the consciousness of the ignorant until you are full of truth; so be loosed into the wilderness and pray that prey is plentiful, so you can eat like a rogue tiger. Young black universe, the likes of you are an endangered species; they kill you off so they can take your organs and examine the very thing that makes you who you are, the melanin. If they could use it for their purpose, they would, because it is magic, and they want to control the magic and break you down into pieces. For your inner peace is what they want to disturb, remember, that should be the least of your worries.

For a conscience opened cannot be shut by any outside entity. Only you can open and close that door, so remember that when they attempt to program you to be something other than what you want to be.

Young black universe, you are a product of the land of the free, so be free to express yourself through your hair, your music, your fashion, the glare is soothing to the caption. Shine as bright as life illuminates your being, for you are a star, super to those who look up to you, they are believing. Your culture is uniting a divided world. Every creed, every race, wants to possess what is natural for you.

Hold your head up so you can see your blessings fall right into your hands. It is hard to see if your head is down, looking up is looking within so you can receive the best of you. You are expanding faster than the speed of light. The enemy aims to slow you down by poisoning the water and food, killing you off with poverty and hunger, and placing you in prison because they cannot stand your might. Just relax and take your place as king of the stars. It is because of you that we are able to produce life for we would not be life if it were not for you and the energy you are. Our young black universe, you are by far the best thing to ever happen to us. We yearn to explore you, attain the riches, and unlock the mysteries of consciousness and time, in a relationship built on trust.

Our young black universe, you are a God, so choose your Goddess on a divine basis and be careful when you mold her consciousness into existence, for a Queen is worthy of master intelligence, so when you fall for her, make sure you fall hard. A family united is a force of Nature, staying united we cannot lose and that's just another reason for them to hate you.

Be careful, Young Black Universe because when they try to destroy the family, they start with the headfirst, every male reduced to nothing and made passive and submissive when our true nature is dominant. When united, we become confident. They know this and to them, I say, "I know the truth hurts." Our Young Black Universe, you are made of melanin and the pineal gland inside the brain produces melanin. It is absolute power, omnipotent in every way to say the same, it is us, my brethren.

Our Young Black Universe, respect your sistas, for their beauty and wit are worthy of respect for the creator, whose beam of light in them has brought love and nurturing for those who choose to kiss her, not diss her. She is your strength and the fuel that makes life work. So, cherish her and do not play with her heart, make sure that her heart does not hurt.

Our Young Black Universe, you are rich and decorated with family. Other stars and planets live within themselves, so do you... I hope this leads to new understandings. You are the absolute of all frequencies, processing information of the cosmos through your cells due to the melanin.

Wake up our Young Black Universe and you can clearly see, this is why you are targeted, because of these powers and abilities. The enemy sees you as a threat because they know of the prophecy and their hate and envy have not weakened. You are young now, but soon you will grow strong and vast. And this confidence of yours will be the only thing that will belong here, it will outlast hate and the test of time.

Many have sacrificed their lives just so I can bring to you this message of hope. But we are redeemed by their bloodshed, so spread this knowledge and these words so that all can see a new Heaven and Earth with the cycling back into power that is happening now, we must keep that dream afloat.

As you keep bringing us into existence, we will continue to show resistance to the few who dare to defy God and set out to control the world when that is not their right. That right belongs to you, Young Black Universe, because it is simply your world. It was in the beginning; it will be in the end. I intend to bring this to you just as it is, Young Black Universe you are the reason we live.

Forgive those who in their ignorance fail to realize the truth that is you, but do not forgive those who see the evidence, and it is right in their face; but they still are angered because they are not you and commence to spurn hate. The enemy is inferior, you are superior, and that truth will ultimately seal their fate.

Remember, when the pressure is on to perform those miracles, it is important for you to understand it's okay to bend, but not break. Education is the key to salvation. The more you know about where you come from, the more you understand about where you are going.

You are the key to creation and this miraculous happening called life is due to your persistent imagination and showing, consistent with all that comes from our contemplations. With you, we are growing. As we grow, I know that these words will glow, providing light for the lost, those of you who have no feelings and cannot elaborate on a thought.

For a thought is the very thing that we are. From your wind, out of your mouth, and into existence, and now here we are. How far do we as a people have to come before we realize that we started this journey? Covering up these truths is a deed that is evil and has come forth to challenge what we believe, so it is the truth that we need to receive and that is what has us yearning.

We are earning the trust of those who are skeptical and are unsure of the rumor that a messiah has come to save us. We have proven that you paid the cost, with all the lives lost to racism, bigotry, and hate. We are redeemed by the bloodshed of our people, and a better new creation awaits us, as we trust that we are the stars, if there is a sequel;

and that the next showing will move the dead and wake us all. For we are in the land of the dead. And we will be that until there is a drastic change in our people.

Young Black Universe, you are our future; thus, you are that change. Commence to aim, aim as high as you can, and let not your dreams for us be destroyed by the beast-like nature and deeds of man. For this new world is your order and divine plan. Where everyone will come to worship, pray, and believe in the same thing.

There is only one truth, and it is all that we know, so show the truth Young Black Universe and let your light continue to glow. We will grow as long as you continue to shine. We are mighty when we think of you, our souls are energized as they begin to incline. In you, we are the sublime, and everything that is between the heights of heaven and the depths of hell is us. We are the gateway to your core, to crossover they have to go through us because we are time.

Our Young Black Universe, let your dreams soar as high as possible, until the unthinkable becomes reality, and the impossible is now possible, even bringing peace to those who are jealous and hostile. You are the bearer of the light, your kingdom is might, so be firm and turn away deceptive imposters. Don't be bothered by those who excrete hate, for their downfall will be that they realize that they fuel your success. Proving them wrong will force them to take their place as you take yours and neutralize. Remember, you are the best. Our

Young Black Universe, these are the words to greatness, place this in your heart because this world belongs to you. So, please put it back in the hands of your originator, the creator, and take it. Our Young Black Universe, these words are from a place that is real, a place within you; so, let them be your foundation and commence to build. The Black Man is the divine essence in all of creation, like the expansion of the universe; so, let your consciousness expand, with no limits to your imagination. Our Young Black Universe, remember who you are, you are the son (sun), and you don't even know that you are a star.

(2012)
TORN BETWEEN HEAVEN & EARTH

They say it is better to have loved once than to have never loved at all. The one time I fell in love it made me believe and feel as if I had never fallen in love at all. As I think back to my traumatic fall from grace, misplaced from the place in which I felt infiniteness in the way of my thoughts being a human entity. As my carnalities take over, I behold the beauty and wonder how my creations have entrapped and embodied my abilities to the point where I have forgotten who I am. But their memory remains. Can it be explained how we got here? *Who or what is God? What is the meaning of the I AM?*

These things I may have misplaced in my memory but my faith in them never misplaced what seems to be an eternity. Some 13. 8 billion years together. But in spirit, we go back even beyond that, thus was the illuminated thought of I AM and what I AM long before my spirit became physical and black and birthed inside a baptism of darkness. As this universe was when it started. As we departed from our originality, which was an infinite thought able to create whatever it wanted, we became apart from its celestial actuality and transformed it into a terrestrial state of being, not of its true reality.

The meta-physical keeps me believing that one day the spiritual can once again be manifested into the physicality, and we are seeing what it is that creates us. *Why were we loved to the point of embodiment and while we are in this physical realm? Why are there energies against us?* One day we will come to know and trust the answer to these questions. But what is it that makes us, is it our soul or our flesh? In the division of the Heavens, a third of the angels fell and merged themselves into physical matter and thus become galaxies, stars, constellations, and planets. By our own understanding, they become us too through our imaginations, coming to us mainly by the passion that created us. Seducing us with that supernatural power until we feel blissfully blessed and have achieved salvation.

And so now since we have merged spirit and the passion, which begets and becomes the flesh, we have life. And a balance of life. Just as soul and flesh, there is positive and negative. For every positive action, there is an equal and opposite reaction, and vice versa. This is the order of the universe or our imagination if you could conceive that kind of contemplation. That our physical consciousness is one with matter and the universe and our flesh is the earth and physical world. As I think greater is she that is in me, than she that is in this world. I wonder about the one inside of me, while thinking about being inside of the one. Then it dawns on me, this is the reason

I fell deep in love in the first place, because neither of them, first the spiritual then the physical could not let me die inside.

For what it is worth, the soul created this consciousness, the universe, and the heavens. They are one, the flesh is a whole other world; I am torn between Heaven and Earth. One to become my wife and the other just to be my girl. The physical Atom. The basic building block of life resides in any entity. Our father, Adham, is light illuminating the universe with his thoughts, his imagination, a woman in the eve, which I have seen in two similar but different beginnings. The infiniteness of spirit and the infiniteness of matter in the physical being. Everything is birthed from one Atom; I do live and believe both ribs are expanding my consciousness. To balance is essential since I gave two parts of me. To create them, their soul is giving way to a whole new thought and now it haunts this. Now those two entities give themselves to conceive and create me. From the physical to the spiritual. In these, I lurk between Heaven and Earth. That is how I am and how I came to be.

(2012)
I AM PLATINUM IN A CITY OF GOLD

I was made different, but my difference is what makes me whole. I realize that because I am unique, I am apart from everything around me, but still within my contraster's soul. As a result of this, I am constantly looked at and viewed as a threat to the rest of the accepted norm because I shine in another way and my thought is different, projecting a different world to you and others as if I am a whole other entity or an alien life form. When the light touches you, you all shine in the same way; the same to say that there is just a golden projection of what was already there, just you. You barely knew that the light that touched you and showed your true color was the color of my complexion. My projection had a gleam to bring the king and queen of creation a reflection of themselves shining like a mirror image. The truth.

So now it seems that you and I are the real proof. There are only the two of us. You were inside of my soul, and I am in yours too. I want you to behold what I am seeing; I am platinum in a city of gold beings. In my soul, a voice is speaking to me, telling me, that I am different and that I should not wish to be like the rest. They are complacent and content with just being full of color, not realizing their full potential, why they were born again and not understanding why they are the best. But to pass the test they must remember why they are the way they are. And not just that they are. As for me, I must believe that my light shines with a difference for a reason; it is meant to attract rather than to become attracted to something that just sees itself instead of the light inside that is blinging.

Beaming, illuminating your soul, covering it like the flesh protecting it because of the covenant with man that together, they mesh like the M.E.S.T. It is as if you embrace that different light, the love of it would not let you see death. In the form of you realizing that you are so unique and now, so special. So much so that I have given you my all, all of my energy to ensure that you reign and live forever, Africa has been bled dry of its diamonds and gold. Collectively, for this country, we have given more than our bodies, we have given our souls; until we have nothing left. There is nothing special about the rest of you which, for you I would take my last breath. Now that I have embraced it here is what the light showed that God was engraved inside my own soul, and I was born platinum in a city of gold.

(2017)
WHAT IS LOVE?

Do we really know what love is, as we all continue through life, will we ever really learn the truth about love? Why it is we live? We live because of the love of mama, even though the drama that goes along with this life we are living can sometimes cause us to forget that the fact of the matter is, we wouldn't know love if it weren't for our mama. Love for ourselves, love for others, or love for just life alone. We would not know these things if it weren't for a mother's love for her family is so strong. We look to the sky above for joyful feelings and peaceful emotions, when in actuality, the reality is that all of those live within us, created by trust from her, believing that you would receive that love and become that love; so that there is no place for a doubtful or hateful notion.

A mother will feed you when you are hungry. She nurtures you when you are sick, she stresses the importance of where you come from so that you'll never forget her. Remember where you come from, the same place that birthed the sky and the stars... A strong, loving, Black woman. Constellation configurations around your mind were designed in her heart. That's just to let you know how powerful you are.

Though she has left the physical world and entered the energetic, spiritual realm, it is this energy when we think of her, her intelligence, her laugh, her sarcastic nature, her genuine concern, and compassion, as we would discuss the emergency which is the sustaining of black life on the planet as it relates biblically. We would talk and she would tell me, "You know that Bible, don't cha!" And I'll be feeling inside, really, I can't hide; it's you bringing out the best in me. And now as love opens up her third eye, we reminisce, and that energy is what brings her back to life.

(2019)
TO THE YOUNG BLACK FEMALE:
OUR YOUNG BLACK UNIVERSE

Our Young Black Universe, take pride in what you have become, Mother to all of creation. Your mind expands wide; engulfing all of our aspirations and connecting us together until we all become one. Without any hesitation, we bow down to your infinite beauty, as we look up to you for our blessings, it is the soul that you possess that soothes me. It is the light and life of every human being, the star, the might in which we gravitate to your sun, or son; the one who will be doing the redeeming.

Our Young Black Universe, life started with you. Remember how powerful you are, as your thoughts expand faster than the speed of light. Your might has traveled as far as the eyes can see. You are the Queen of existence, carry yourself appropriately, that way the enemy will respect you and will find difficulty in showing his resistance. Take pride in being dark. For inside the darkness contains beautiful entities within, all rich with natural resources, enough to cure the world of poverty. Make every being rich again. Your Blackness is rich like oil, the melanin protects you from any kind of harm.

Powered by the rays of the sun, it is feeding you information about yourself and the cosmos every second by second. It is connecting you back to where you come from, the original source, and that source is the force from where we came, also known as the omnipotent one. Embrace your dark beauty, my love. For your physical build is the reason those stars rotate and spin. Just as the mind of boys to men who are captivated by your beauty.

This is the reason you are a Goddess, and our pride as mortal men is shaken, when you awaken the energies inside of us as the light reveals the truth about the darkness. We as your opposite realize now who started this. It was an immaculate miraculous conception. The dividing of one Atom or Adam into two. Just as the Eve, you are the one entity that all of the stars travel through. You have to believe. Believe in yourself, our Young Black Universe that you can entice us to look to you, the sky to see our blessings. For if our heads are held low to the ground, it's virtually impossible to see them fall, pound by pound. Thus, we continue stressing. Never be ashamed of who you are, where you come from, or how you look because the Good Book states that you, the kingdom, is arrayed in fine linen and that you are full of riches of untold wealth.

Knowing these things ahead of yourself serves as medicine for your spiritual health. And it is the reason I will continue to show you these gifts. So, you continue to have breath as breath means soul or spirit. It means consciousness, to say the least. Our Young Black Universe, remember why I was conceived. To bring to my kind the truth about the riches of the Kingdom, to stabilize this violent, chaotic universe and bring to it peace.

Please, my child, embrace every part of your Blackness. Your melanin is powerful. You are a lot stronger than you know. The world lives inside of you. There are things about it that you need to know. At this present time, it is a male-dominated society. But before, my Young Black Universe, the divine feminine once ruled the planet. There is a new day dawning, it is your time now my Young Black Universe to assert your dominance. Women are becoming empowered all over the globe, we need that. Your nurturing and healing power our Earth, is being destroyed not by women but by greedy old men who cannot let go. Our Young Black Universe, please reveal to me all of your mysterious secrets so that I may return home with them and remember why you wanted us to keep it. Please believe it when I say that you are Queen of Queens. Your majestic swagger is pure royalty, and your aura is like something out of a dream.

Our Young Black Universe, everything revolves within you. You are special to the point to where God is completely focused on you. Waiting to reveal your beautiful soul to the world and extend to us another truth as we transition into the next dimension. This is what I see in you. Multi universes, each one a different reflection of you. You are our mother nature, and the enemy wants to divide and conquer the Black family. You are the family. That is the reason they hate you. Keep on doing you, showing your style, showcasing your swagger, which is the way to have the entire world following you to life in the hereafter. There are 12 astrological signs after your 12 cycles that you have as a woman, just as the 12 cycles of our moon.

The sun travels through each cycle in the course of a year, bringing light to each sign. We live in the womb here on Earth just waiting to be born again, so there is no fear of dying. Our Young Black Universe, do not be ashamed of your hair, for your hair is your culture, and now other races are aware. Never be ashamed of where you come from, for Africa is the richest continent on the planet. Your wisdom is gold, and your blood is oil. So, see how wealthy you are in resources. The enemy is doing everything he can to get you off course and go and get to the riches, and spoils, and they will damn any trace of you. So, my Young Black Universe, be wise, never look past what is in front of you.

Right now, there is a war on women. All across the Middle East, United States, China, etc. There has been a need by man to destroy what is best for you. These words are what is best for you. Never settle for less than what you deserve. For you are Heaven and Earth and you should be treated like royalty. You are the epitome of a Goddess whose presence commands man's attention and loyalty, as you make him the proudest. Before the foundation was laid, there was the soil… see.

Now we roar the loudest because we know who came in order before thee. Our Young Black Universe, you are dancing to the Earth's heartbeat. Please continue to move, it is the most beautiful thing in existence. Just us watching you, my soul is soothed and as we continue to groove, every soul will get loose and reminiscent. Our vibe does prove efficient that there is a God in you. Our Young Black Universe, your beauty is our pride, and that is something we use for healing. To peace, love, happiness, and soul, your womb is where power resides; and to that, we will forever be true. Let us let the light glow, because without you, nothing would be living.

(2020)
CHANNELING

Over 400 years of oppression, ancestors were beaten, murdered, and raped. Hate never seemed to cease its progressions, for so many never seemed to see a better day. In 2021, we still seem to have issues with race. On the one hand, they hate us for being dark, on the other hand they have embraced our culture. Be that as it may, they may want to start a race war; I say a holy war is what it will turn out to be. And that's what it will take, once true Israel is recognized as a people with a black face and a people with circumcised hearts. The reason for all of the hate? The truth can be quite dismantling and so for that reason alone, I am forever channeling our ancestors' dreams, from the beginnings of the universe to the future of the mind and heart.

I see you when I look up into the sky. The warmth and the light activate my melanin and vigor for life. I seek potential mates in order to procreate and continue to be fruitful and multiply. I do not partake in anything that would cause me to hate another person's blessing before mine.

I want to be dwelling in the land you create for me. Flowing with milk and honey, rich with materials, creating the spiritual with days of blessings added on and on for the centuries of stressing over the bloodshed of our ancestry.

You engineered humanity. Though you may be from another galaxy, I can feel your being getting closer and closer until there is nothing left but a new reality. Now I know where my place is, in between you and the earth. Since before the earth, my race had its place here, over, and over. When you arrive into this solar system, I am the Black conscious that you must rebirth. I never lean to my own understanding. I close my eyes. It is your spirit and word I partake in first, then everything else I see I am channeling. Into the deep of the abyss, I jump in headfirst. The kingdoms and governments are what I intend to be dismantling as I am channeling negative and positive energies from the sun, through us and within us, upon, and around the Earth. I am channeling the sun's (son's) energy, warmth, and word into your ears. Tell me what you hear, what you heard. If in your thoughts my presence is near, we are power, because knowledge and wisdom are here. Then do not fear, we have merged.

(2020)
INTERSTELLAR

As you look amongst the stars, you become one with the space between them. You close your eyes, replace them with an inner vision, and then you see all of our solar system from afar. Every planet you visited, there was no need to leave them. Each one feels like home. It is just another place for your soul to roam. As you sit back and think, *What are they on and how could they ever explore you? Do they believe that they can destroy you?* However, you live forever. You are interstellar. You are the space between stars, they realize that, when they try to travel through you. For you are chaotic, without order, you are lord. You are free and there is nothing that can subdue you. You see that your dark skin is one with the darkness of the universe. Behold. You are the mystery.

I never knew you till now... remember me? They think hard before they try to remember us, and how it starts. First with circumcised hearts, then we will break the curse. They knew that before they ever knew you. Radiation from the sun, our inner being will wake the dead, the nation of dark-complected beings because of all the bloodshed of our ancestors, those who kept the sacred teachings to give you. We are light beings, beaming brightly through life, like the sun, or son, before us. Our pigment is embedded into the blackness of the universe, how clever. We are forever and that is why they come after us, thanks to that notion, through space we are coasting like a thunderbird. Will you stop moving? No. Never. Your mind glides in the ever. They try to kill you, they may never. The enemies plan, we sever, however, because you and me, together are interstellar.

(2020)
OUT IN ORBIT

There is no limit to the height of my consciousness, and for the endangered Black man. There is no limit to the extermination of our kind. But my mind continues to rise in the midst of the slaughtering, slicing back with words from the word, a language in which we all know, and I can accelerate in a rhyme. The long haul, huh, well I have been here for it. I am out in orbit, conversing with beings of another kind. They tell me to wait a minute before I unleash the nuclear bomb, exposing the core of the planet right before my enemy's eyes. They say some of them are starting to get it, realizing that we are the only way to the prize, into the riches and wealth. Be wise.

Their envy and hatred grow with each passing decade; are you surprised? They want to bring us to death and attain our God-given riches and wealth; leaving us desolate and naked, knowing nothing of whom we are or how we used to be in this land before time; and knowing nothing of our throne or our God-like minds. This is the level I am on, whatever hate you throw at the black sky, I have proven I am too high… I cannot hate, so I absorb it. Yeah, remembering how

I got to this place, stepping on giants until the rest of the evil in them forfeited. Look up, haters, you see, we, me, and my people, are out in orbit.

(2020)
RESURRECTED

What are races when every race and creed originated from one source? One truth became affected before we knew that there was a lie. Do we really die, or breathe another substance in another body on another planet in another galaxy? Does greed intervene with the thrill of living life or are we content to just stay rested? Here is what I invested, into the hearts of the deities. Whether you believe we are one or that we all may not be. I believe that race was created to separate and divide, to conquer the masses of the people who are really of one tribe; whose true king is someone from another life and made visible in this dimension through stories of heroes and messiahs who made incredible sacrifices and come to save us. We are the saviors. In the same way that we make like the solar system, we are embodied planets, and we plan it out. We leave no doubt about whatever else was expected. I am going to present this life to the next with gratefulness to ensure my being gets a new life, my soul, a star resurrected.

(2020)
THE POETIC DIALECT
OF SCHIZOPHRENIA

I suffer from this crazed disease. Audio and visual hallucinations. I see what I hear and hear what I see. I believe I am a product of my meditation, and so in order to conceive a life where there is nothing more but imagination, I have been able to foresee my right to exist and to lay claim to this great nation, built off of the blood of my ancestry. In my mind I fight for my own salvation as if I were a roaring beast not a human being, sinking my teeth into the flesh of bigotry and racism.

I rip out the heart of doubt in its conscience and prey on their next move while they try to assassinate my character because they cannot understand me. They say that I do not make sense, that I have distorted thoughts. I see, believe, and hear things that are not there or that are not true.

To me, that sounds like something lost. These seven voices I hear in my head are God, so why should I listen to you? The struggle with this life that I have had, has been very hard, and another level of difficulty, especially when everyone is blind and void. I am the only one who can see the truth. Lucifer and God merged into one person, the same lord, this is just my personality, the you in me and the me in you. Everything has a positive and/or negative charge.

Good and Evil, that is our actuality. A life without one of those two sides is not a life; for there is no reality for life… there would be no proof. For we could not know one without experiencing the other.

How could the universe exist without the darkness of night, the woman, and man, the light of the stars, they are the forever eternal lovers. We only need those two. Schizophrenia used to be known as something demonic. An inner-dimensional power in which the church cannot explain the reason for the demon, so that's my reason to jump on it. I attempt to maintain, regardless of if I can or not; but the seasons will continue to change, and change starts with what is in the heart and that's my part in all of this.

Before it drives the world insane, I'll take blame for the reason. Fire, I don't run from it. My name, Timothy V. Lane, I am a Schizophrenic. After this piece, bring peace and remember how to play the game. Don't ever think that you can't win it. The end, I am running towards it. With this communication with Heaven, we all never meant to offend you. Our imagination speaks, and spreads forever. This is the Poetic Dialect of Schizophrenia. This is my truth.

(2020)
THE POETIC DIALECT OF
SCHIZOPHRENIA (PART 2)

As I sit back and listen to the voices in my head, they tell me "Be patient," and wait your turn, because when you turn, the powers that be will burn inside a glorious light, a sight to see until they are spiritually dead." Just as the Israelites have been for thousands of years. We search around blinded, praying for a light, but we cannot find it. We are lost in the darkness of night held captive but blinded by our ancestors' blood, sweat, and tears.

So many of us suffer from post-traumatic slave syndrome, multigenerational trauma, and injustice. So many of us never found our way home because the lord in whom we believed had become our enemy. No longer could we love it, with no life love, just dead hate in the form of a white messiah who was a fake and the symbol of white supremacy, the reason we could not trust it.

Fast forward some 400 years later, they still remain to be our number one haters. The slave masters and the KKK reside at the police stations. They traded in their hoods and sheets for batons, tasers, and guns and they claim to keep the peace as they aim and shoot first before we can turn and run, and they ask questions later, to say the least. With all of this going on and then I have to worry about whether you are going to divide my family and home, brainwashing my kids in the classroom and even worse when they are home, with your social media, television, and radio tones.

The poisoning of our food and water is just too much to dwell on. Life is a game to be played, and I am glad I'm playing it. Given that a lot of times, it can be overwhelming; the beauty of it all is that I see things as a Schizophrenic, and in that is where I'm dwelling.

(2021)
WE THE PEOPLE

We the people, the foundation of this great nation. We the people yearn to be treated as equals and not treated and seen as the lesser, but that we become greater than our oppressors and the only way to true salvation. That vision of that great super nation.

Where we the people show precision in laying the blueprint and foundation for all nations and governments all over the world. The feeling of utopia, peace be unto you my real ancestor, Cush; Ethiopia. You don't see how or why he created the sky, sun (son), and moon, from the Black woman's womb. My roots run deep, and rampant like the creation of my favorite girl.

The world I thought I showed Eve was at the golden time of day, call it heaven, the throne of the son (sun) sets forever, and we have shown that we believe and that we can brighten another day. A Mahogany flame burns on because we the people grow strong, electing our leaders who pass laws that affect the world today.

Our right to vote is the one power that they cannot suppress. We the people built this nation on blood, sweat, tears and death. They want

to take us to a dark place. On the dollar, it says "In God We Trust."
If we want to see Black economic wealth flourish, we gotta have faith
in that… we must. Lord, forgive us because we cannot seem to
conquer evil, we need more than a savior now, we need, "we the
people."

(2021)
AM I THE ONLY ONE
SEEING THIS? (PART 1)

Thinking about my life and how it came to be 6 protons, 6 neutrons, 6 electrons, the carbon atom or Adam. Sunlight shining through man, the star in the dark of the beast. At least that's how they made it to be when I read those twenty-two chapters: in the end, the revelation told me that it was me. I damn near fell to my face when I heard them speak and say to me "You see," as I continued to read, "it's you. You are the reason for this universe, this kingdom to be."

I asked them, "But what about the 400 years of slavery?" Then they answered with *Genesis 15:13* and I quote what it spoke as God spoke to Abraham and said, "Know for certain that for 400 years, your descendants will be strangers in a country and land not their own, and that they will be enslaved and mistreated there. I will punish the nation they serve as slaves and afterward, they will come out with great possessions."

So, with that I have to ask ISRAEL, Are you ready for this?" The reason that they proceed to kill us is because we are cursed but still, they feel as if it heals us to be rebirthed in the name of a white Messiah, Jesus. Zeus never seemed to be able to reveal us; but he took credit for the salvation and creation of a zealous and resilient nation; it hurts, Israel, *Black people, what is this? How can we get back to euphoric bliss? Is this my imagination? Am I the only one seeing this?*

(2021)
AM I THE ONLY ONE
SEEING THIS? (PART 2)

What about the year 1978? The Meek were birthed and would inherit the Earth. I too was born, and the strong will lead the reborn to a new day. A place of Utopia and when I learned of the might of the son of Ham, Cush Ethiopia, I prayed we would not be slaves because we had hope in you every step of the way.

It seems that we came from kings and queens and all that is divine. It is also a remnant of my mind. When I dream, I realize that there were two others of my kind, also born in the year 1978. A Leo in August and a Virgo in September. As I remember our paths crossed twenty years later and I am still amazed today. Two heavens playing one game inside my mind. But I wasn't ready to be a player, at least not at that time, anyway. There was a lock on my heart and on the other hand, I pimped my pin. I am the son though we were all a part, we were one.

To be spiritually connected was the intention then. We all three graduated in 1996. There go those sixes again, like at the beginning of this piece that I first mentioned. It seemed meant to be. I guess the Messiah was meant to be a p.i.m.p. I believed in G.O.D. being a D.O.G was not where I had my attention.

Two heaven stars in the lone star state, in the city of the star where Dallas, Texas is the landmark of the lord. We do things big in Texas, is a saying that stretches as big as the state. And it is euphoric bliss. With all of this that I have pointed out to you, I ask you, am I the only one seeing this?

(2021)
AM I THE ONLY ONE
SEEING THIS? (PART 3)

On a quest to expand my conscious knowledge and wisdom, I was in school looking for someone to woo and share my vision. As I began to travel through that day on the train from school, it was then that I saw my chance. At first glance, the average man would not think about it or either have a bad intention. However, I am not an average man. I was excited, even flabbergasted. She was even more gorgeous. Did I mention sitting alone? I went to sit right next to her and I felt right at home. I wanted to know what she thought about us and if she was, in fact, thinking about it. You could say it was either love or lust, a lie or trust.

To be truthful about it, her fragrance heightened my senses in a way that only the sun can. I just wanted to be her man and it really was more about love than lust. I asked her what she was wearing. She spoke softly but sternly and said, "Egyptian Musk" and from then on, I knew it was God's plan.

That was in 2003, fast forward 18 years later and you will see we are now realizing that Egypt is responsible for all of our agricultural, scientific, mathematical, and economic knowledge. Mahogany, my queen to be. This world is yours and forever will I be. I think of what you mean to me, more than the sun and the moon. Your presence forever looms over all who try and cause the chosen's downfall, if you cannot love me, then who can? My Mahogany Byrd, sweet and bitter at the same time as the earth. You are an angel. You take flight with might and bliss, in between the heavens. I have to ask, am I the only one seeing this? This is forever.

(2021) ANNIVERSARY
(FOR MOM AND DAD)

Anniversaries are a simple reminder of what constitutes the creation of God. The vows you made on this day made you one flesh and all of this mess, the stress, years later it's just a test and another way to strengthen your hearts. Remember what about you got you this far, the anticipation of true love blossoming, divine meditations of what it would be like to be together forever. Your thoughts for each other intertwine, following the lord's calling of love and light in the dark. No matter what you think it means, many years later, you were brought together for a reason. Now, 'tis the season to get rid of the hatred hater; hate inside destroys you with pride. Too big to admit that you were vulnerable without each other. You need the confirmation in your lives. At this point whatever it is that you decide, know that I (we) am the product of your love. You two together inside of me can never die. Before I wrote this, I said a prayer to the Lord above,

Dear Lord, let them remember why they love each other so,
let them realize that they are each other's souls. No matter
what they have been through in the past, at least on this day,
Lord, let them celebrate it religiously, because in love they

may not get another chance. Right now, they think that they are adversaries, but on the contrary, they are best friends, and we want to wish them many more happy anniversaries.

Yours truly,

Timothy and family

(2021)
AS I HUG A DEMON IN THE LIGHT
AN ANGEL KISSES ME IN THE DARK

How could I not feel God's might, when everyone that I touch is a divine spark? Here is a new twist to the plight. We showcase how we feel about our lord. Our souls give him the strength to fight, and even with that, the fact is to get the win, it is still hard. For our enemy is formidable against us, how long will we be oppressed? They think we were destined to be slaves; they are the ones who are really corrupt while we hope to be blessed.

There is one who humbles them; when they organize and act up with more or maybe less, He will save the day. We pray to someone to relieve our stress. We don't know if it is pagan or not, because every religion derived from one source. There is only one way. The truth is now lost inside of our enemy's plot. The only way to retrieve it, melanin play. It plays a key role in this universe's existence. In this the galaxy's secret we can unlock. And take back this world by teaching the truth about life, man and woman, husband and wife, who created today.

As I hug a demon in the light, an angel kisses me in the dark. While this side of this world has my soul tonight, my melanated flesh is the other side and thrives off of the sun rays and that gives me might.

We pray to be in your presence, to do that with ourselves we have to fight, a tussle for and with our souls so that one day, we can grow and then we can see the sun at midnight. In our ability to do that, we become the lord. We are full of grace and power showered with divine blessings because our ancestors had it so hard.

(2021)
CONVERSATIONS WITH
ME AND MYSELF

Myself: Hey, what up, bro? You look down. What's wrong?

Me: Oh, I don't know. With all that is happening right now. I am a little confused. I feel like I'm lost. I've been gone.

Myself: Lost as in trying to make it home?

Me: I guess you could say that. But not the kind of home you think. I'm not talking about a home like that.

Myself: A home is a home, don't you think; one you bought?

Me: A home is a shell protecting what is within, from what is above and below. To be in sync with everything without a shell is a home of thought.

Myself: Oh, that's deep, bro. What direction are you going when you begin to travel to this place?

Me: I ask myself that a million times. Where are we headed in this world today? So much depends on race; and if not that, how much I make, or if I could be bought.

Myself: Ok, I see where your mind is. Your mind is in another state. You think outside of the box, where there is no relation between distance and time. There is no embodiment, no shackles, or locks. There is nothing to limit your being in just one place. You are an eternal thought, which is sublime. With that in mind, how could you feel lost? All you have to do is be confident and sure about who you are. Be aware of your surroundings and space.

Me: That's good advice. Tell me, how did you get so smart? That was heartfelt.

Myself: I had an epiphany one day and it was outstanding. I think I might be, Lord, because I had a conversation with me and myself.

A Dedication to
Malcom X and Martin Luther King, Jr.

(2021)
GOOD CUSH, SEX AND CONVERSATION

I push until she flexes her sex, so I increase the stimulation and then I begin with her imagination. The contemplation, the creation of the movement of the sun and the sea, and my soul united with the state of her body. This is Sacred Eternal Xtasy. We are burning stars intertwined in a binary orbit with one another, providing a double light, so that other couples can see and absorb it and then become lovers.

Good cush, sex, and conversation. Girl, you say that's something that you never get. Niggaz always use you for your physicality instead of penetrating your soul the way I would, once I had your imagination lit. Getting it good and hot, in actuality, sizzling hot and steaming, we intertwine our thoughts and become pure light, until our bodies are one and we start high beaming.

Once we are lit, we take a few hits and then we are able to take a look into each other's soul. We drift in and out of other dimensions together but then there are three in which the bliss is the pinnacle.

And it is the pinnacle in which we go. When you cum, we both turn into gold and then it follows us everywhere, every place that we go. The bright gold light of wisdom oozes from our being, blinding those who are dumbfounded and ignorant of the plan.

See it's the master plan that moves us to master the universe through the African ghetto karma sutra. So, relax, relate, release, lie down right here or take a seat, whatever suits ya. We are about to blast off, get off, if that is what soothes ya. From my lungs to my tongue through to your soul and back and forth we go. We ride each other's brain waves; they take us coast to coast. Good cush, sex, and conversation are something that I provide. Mind sex creates the astral plane. Now it's your time to come and get this. It is our salvation.

In this, I don't boast, but come and enjoy a ride.

(2021)
HE IS BEING CRUCIFIED
AS WE SPEAK

Thinking of how we came to be. Poverty and slavery made him too strong for them to control. See? They captured him in us, then nailed him/us to a cross for the followers to see. All because he/we proclaimed ourselves to be, more than what they are, we proclaimed to be Lord, as we the people create Christ's body. The morning star as the word Christ originates from the word "Christos," referencing the compacting together of melanin, black on black coming together crystalizing into pure light, the might of the star, and light of the son (sun). How far have we really come, when the beatings still continue and the bloodshed flows from a beating heart giving in, living inside of a beast, as the Atom birthing the universe in the dark.

Get it? I hope you do, because this that I reveal to you will be proof. Proof of how Christianity has enslaved us too. Then made us the very thing that we pray for, death, they want us deceased. Zeus is death. Jezeus never breathed a breath. In the image of a slave master, a white Messiah, we found more pain and heartache because of what that image left. Our feet, pierced, and pinned to a cross so that we cannot stand on our own. Our hands, pierced with nails, we feel every bit of hell because we fail to use them to build for the future generations. How will they prevail, what will they become? And to top it all off, they placed a crown of thorns upon our cranium so we cannot think straight and so that we make mistakes when we try to free ourselves and take aim at them.

For centuries, they used the story of Jesus not to build us up, but rather to let us know that, no matter how much we think we are above the hold and try to unite, their main goal and intention is to divide, conquer, and destroy us and show that any hope of a Black united nation in their world must go. That flame, we can ignite. Christianity has enslaved us on so many levels. How do we really know for sure that we are worshipping God? What if you are worshipping the devil? So many hypocritical Christians believe that they are of the prince of peace; unknowingly, not recognizing that bloodshed is how you get peace and how to advance to the next level. Wake up, Black people, the only way to get peace is to cleanse the land with the blood of our enemies. Then you, and me, will be free. You have to be willing to die for it. See? He is being crucified as we speak.

(2021)
KREATION: TO MY MOTHER, HAPPY BIRTHDAY

On this day, you were brought into this world, to the proud parents; C.L. and Sarah. A beautiful, melanated goddess, an infinite infant baby girl. It was easy to see when you were young and free that in this life, you were not a novice; it was like you had been here before. A queen to be, you are nature to me. Your dominating presence can't go unnoticed, it's obvious, it's a water hole for us to drink, leaving us satisfied and thirsty no more. I think, *what else, lord, do you have in store?* You taught me that the core of understanding was understanding that at the core of existence is our imagination, made possible through your birth on this day. I pray, and I am amazed by the kreation.

Now understanding my contemplations of how I came to be, how we came to be, let it be our mother who buys back the plantations. So that we can exercise the demons who continue with false accusations, in hopes of deteriorating you and me and our current situations. Mother, your teachings are my salvation. That I will never forget. Our adaptation to the climate is like cremation. With that, I know our future is bright and lit, providing light for another night and future generations to carry on what you started with your kids. Today is a day of celebration, because of this day I live to see my kreation. It is them that I continue to will. Happy birthday, mom, this is the gift that I can give. I love you.

(2021)
ON THE OUTSIDE FROM WITHIN

On the outside from within. When you stop thinking, that's when I begin. I stay true to the teachings, but you lie about sin. What are we to believe if we cannot put our trust in him? Why were we created? If it was done out of love, then why are we hated? Were we created to be slaves in the first place? Why were we programmed to only use 10% of our brain? Working to save you from the labor, I asked the maker: is it dominance that you are out to attain? Is this what you call amazing grace?

The Gnostics taught that we, unknowingly, worship the evil one. The demiurge who created himself and the angels and demons out of nothing, the womb of feminine darkness. So, it really comes down to whom the people want. It was the immaculate conception. It's dark in here, hold up! I'm getting ready to spark this. The angels were created to keep order in this prison for souls which we call the universe. Now I see why the Hebrews and Black people are made to suffer, it's cold, and they're cursed. I guess that's what really hurts. If our creator is evil, tell me, what is life really worth? Well, we have a soul, and that is gold. It's what good and evil really want to control, for in that, is power on Earth. So, ask yourself, what do you believe and who do you believe in? I think back as I sit back and relax, thinking about the son (sun) the one, as we begin, the rebirth of our souls, it grows on the outside from within.

(2022)
PUPPETS & THE PUPPET MASTERS

We have gotten to a point where we have learned from our oppressors how to enslave and suppress or oppress our own thoughts. We express that we are free physically, but we have become slaves mentally, distressed, and depressed. Why can't we free ourselves from the strings of what our enemies taught?

On so many levels they have tried to control our minds and the way that we think. They realize that the power of our perception can keep them alive, away from certain self-destruction because they know that they are on the brink. We don't think or use our own intuition or our imaginations. We allow what we perceive through the media and society to think for us. We get trapped inside that thought and cannot free ourselves from the situation. Our minds are influenced by programming from television and radio. What we hear and what we see is what we believe to be.

We cannot receive the visions and the sounds of the inner world which constitutes the divinity of our soul. Social media now has us all under mind control. Obsessed with politics, relationships, race, religion, and economics instead of what is truth. Knowledge and wisdom are the streets of gold. This is me and you. So preoccupied with phones, Iphones, and Androids. Why can't we tune into the vibrations of the universe, so we cannot be played with like toys.

Puppets don't speak by themselves. The puppet master makes their noise. The truth is, we have all become toys. Because of all this we are distracted and can't be in tune with or connect to a higher intelligence. That is the sole basis of being here; to be in tune with nature and the order of the universe, not to have our imaginations assassinated because of our own negligence. I feel like if I didn't write this, it would be negligent, so I would be headed for disaster. Now what becomes of the hereafter? Have we become irrelevant in a world of puppets controlled by those puppet masters?

(2021)
TRAVELING THROUGH THE GALAXY
- THE SEXTRA-TERRESTRIAL

I am traveling through the galaxy in a place somewhere beyond the sun. A search to stimulate your sexuality has begun, a sexual mission, a trip to the depths of our souls. As we unearth the vision, Mercury will be the first rendition, a release of the unborn. No life, no atmosphere, heavy breathing on here. Are you to be my wife, or not? We travel to the second tier, a planet whose sex is fierce, administrating rain on a regular. Sulphuric acid is her vagina's tears. She delivers O G's here. Violent, volcanic passion erupts in her. Every time her mountains quiver, lava flows from her body because she knows the dictations here. As we relate, we have mind sex, dirty talk telepathically as we speak without speaking; controlling body language as her body quakes and we both came extremely close to the zenith.

Speaking is believing and seeing is believing. And for what that's worth, for the first time I see the whole Earth. It is so beautiful it hurts but not as violent as her twin sister, Venus. I am leaving her now, dwelling' in the third. Now I can inhibit my freaky nature into these bodies and beings and have them do whatever the hell I want them to do. Because of their fascination with the fire and my word, now I can give you the world and if you desire, the other planets too.

What you heard was the truth, the fame, my name, and how I relate to you and pray you through this alien karma sutra, and into the game. With our souls groovin, shiiiit, now men and women rule everythang. I am a whole host of heavenly, intellectual, sexuals. The anticipation of your orgasm, I can maintain, just clinch me when you are ready to let yourself loose and bust. Trust your soul, mind, and body with I.

I am the SEXTRA-TERRESTRIAL, Mr. Love to lust, Timothy V. Lane

(2021)
SISTER

We were born in the same year, and a little bit over a month apart. I feel like we were twins who had different fears, but still here for whatever reason, we never left our connectors' heart. Our father who art in Heaven, hallowed, be thy name, our father who created the Earth. Rest assured our mothers, who are like Heaven and Earth, are one in the same.

Ms. Meek today is the day you become stronger than our creator, your soul, like your skin, is pure gold shining bright because of the flaming light that is me, your brother, the sun (son), because of us they trust, and people now can see. Some of them love us but most of them are haters. The meek shall inherit the Earth and the strong shall lead. God did not come late, He just decided to delay us and waited til just the right time to reveal the King and Queen of what it is to be.

My dear Ms. Meek, you will own the world one day; even if it comes through the next generation, our children will make the way. Just pray and be thankful for all that you are, a perfect combination of power and beauty with the intelligence to raise a nation. I thank our Father for this day.

You are my better half and I just want to add that you will no longer worry one day, and it starts with me wishing you a very happy birthday.

Sincerely,

Tim

(2020)
THANKFUL

I sit here today with all of the failures and disappointments of the human race, with just a day to propel and tell you of a future anointment of what it means to be in God's grace. We often live life, taking it for granted while we are young. Only to feel later that life was just handed to us for a short while. It takes that long to finally understand it, and we do once we are gone. So, while I have the chance, I want to say to God, "Thank you!"

The only way that I can advance is to acknowledge the truth in you. That becomes and overcomes me to where I must take a stance with the proof that I see, the way you have blessed me. You are my Lord. Though I may not see it from the whole perspective, I must thank you for what I can see, for all of my imperfections, and for what I cannot see. I walk by faith, not by sight, until I can feel my way around the deep, dark night, until I can feel the blessing. So, from here on out, there is no room for stressing because I thank you for all that we as a people are going through. I know that true power and grace are nothing but mere reflections of what we can say that we are, as a united people.

We, the greater of two evils, will champion a cause as colossal as you are GOD yourself, and unity will be a strong formidable force amongst the people, with good trumping over evil, as we exit this life and enter the sequel. The Next Life After Death. I will say I am thankful even with my last breath, even when I am old and feeble.

(2021)
THANKFUL (PART 2)

I am thankful for my life, and life within itself. Also, for my wife and my children, for every time you breathe, I know they have breath. We are living in a crazy chaotic world.

But still, I thank you Lord GOD, if for nothing else, the creation of it, which was done when the guy found his girl. Never could I have imagined a place with such beautiful scenery. I stare at a supermoon and then the stars at night, they seem to be staring back, hypnotizing my soul, at least that is what that means to me.

I feel the breeze and then as I hear the wind, I focus in on the beauty of the grass and trees. What we need is in form of the beauty of the sun which produces the most valued vitamin D. Bright rays that I pray would increase my melanistic power, so that I can be the brawn and dawn of a new day and century while becoming the man of the hour.

I thank you GOD for my mother and father, and my sister who work together to keep me grounded; so that I don't get beyond myself and do something to hurt my prowess. I am not dumbfounded to the point where I'm powerless. I realize that our prize is flawless, and we become that once we realize we are not slaves, that in our minds it has been abolished. So, now let's attain wealth. Be Thankful if for nothing else, because of your life. For we all must see death because what will be left will not be right.

(2021)
THE FUTURE
HAPPENED YESTERDAY

The future happened yesterday. Today is a reflection of what happened in the past. Tomorrow is the result of what happened today, so that we will not forget how far we have come, being that we once were first, but now in society, we are last. Once, the Alpha; more dominant than our creators' past. We were the future and manifestation of the Almighty. Then we fell from that grace because we wanted the future to happen today, without preparing for an all-nighter just to see tomorrow, which we should have been doing yesterday.

Now you can say we need a minute, and this moment was at its very last. I pray to God that you don't come too late because we need you in this, if for nothing else than for their sake to let the future know that this and these times too, will all pass. Scripture says the last will be the first and the first will be the last. There is nothing new under the sun (son), and I guess what they say is true. The past, the present, and the future are all happening now at the same time as one, just as when we all pray. We won, wake up now. Not only are we the Alpha, but we are also the Omega. The beginning and the end, at least that's what the words say. This is the beginning of the end, because the future happened yesterday.

(2021)
THE GREATEST FEELING I EVER FELT
(A TRIBUTE TO MY FOUR DAUGHTERS)

The greatest feeling I've ever felt was holding you for the first time. When I first saw you, I knew you were mine. Not just because of your resemblance to your mother and me, but the light that shined through you was so bright, I felt like, *how could I ever leave you? How could I ever die?* When I held you close to me, you were so warm at night. I prayed to God to forgive me for my past transgressions and that He would open your mind up to full capacity so you would be happy intertwining with all of your blessings, having great insight. Partaking in his love and might.

If there ever is a plight by our enemies to destroy you, I will sniff it out like the lion that I am and destroy it and them with my paws with one swipe. They might seek you because you seek truth. I am with you even until the end of the world. You are the proof. I know for sure that there is a God. His heart beats inside my beautiful, genius baby girls. Don't ever let anyone tell you that you can't achieve and pay attention and let me mention. Don't let any man fail you or make you think that you cannot believe. You are a future queen. But for right now you are a princess. My princesses, call on me if you should ever need my help. Because having you was the greatest feeling that I have ever felt.

(2021)
MOTHER'S DAY

I wish I could undo all of the hurt. Over the years, I have realized your worth. More valuable than life itself, the power you possess as a Black woman will raise us from our spiritual death.

Even though to release these feelings I have struggled with myself, remember mom, you showed me what was important in life, the good treatment and respect owed to women is the reason why I have attained spiritual wealth.

I owe all that I am and that I dream to be to your teachings, remembering those things you taught me and even though it is hard, in God I am still believing.

I wish I could retire you and send you on a vacation around the world. It is because of you my mother that I have been able to love another, thus Mahogany, only with you too mother, becomes my favorite girl.

Although I don't have money to shower you with gifts like you deserve, I hope that you feel important to us, because it lifts our confidence up when you are soothed from our words.

Trust me mother when I say that one day you will get the credit that belongs to you for birthing this, our Young Black Universe. The grace is heaven's throne for you, for your faith in God, which was not shaken, even though we lost so many, we never feared the worst.

And with that I want to say thank you for all of the education, quality time, and fun. We just want to wish you a Happy Mother's Day in this year 2021.

(2021)
THE TREE OF LIFE

In between the Heaven and Earth stands a tree. Reaching high into the sky, conversing with the heavens about you and me. We are connected from beneath the earth as our roots do run deep. Praise be to the most high, because I am blessed to be poetically inclined to try to describe this vision, giving life to this artistic piece.

Energy from the sun and rain to the seed was sent back by the growth of the tree and continues to be why I aim to be the one who can climb to the top, realizing that the sublime cannot be stopped. I am never alone because I am connected by the root up to the crown, and there is nothing that can keep me bound as I begin to leave the ground climbing all the way up.

A tree connects the heaven, the earth and the underworld all together with the branches reaching towards the sky. It is a symbol of man's perpetual yearning to become more than life while his roots keep him grounded and connected to the Earth's core and light. Dreaming of how high I can reach, I keep climbing until I can see nothing but the sun shining. Then with the subtle breeze, the leaves of the tree speak and say to me "If you continue to seek, then you will continue to keep finding. The root of who you are is at the root of the universe. The Atom's light, God's might show through the rhyming of each poetic verse."

The fruits are ripe on the family tree of life. Never forget the tree's worth.

(2021)
WALKIN' THROUGH THE VALLEY
OF THE SHADOW OF DEATH

I am walking through the valley of the shadow of death, I hear screaming voices in the dark; it makes me wonder if I have taken my last breath. Am I another spark created from a star that is too hot and too far for me to reach back to? I give whatever is left of me, then preach, and teach how I got that far without being brought to the reality that what I see may be my imagination too. In actuality, hallucinations, I have felt for as long as I have been aware that I can feel.

Myself and the voices are even, so I guess this life that we experience is even kill. Still though, I live on. I am just hoping that one day I will make it to the light and become that. That light, eventually taking my place on my father's throne. I hope I can find my way home. Thy rod and staff are supposed to comfort me, but I feel weaponless. You are just leaving my soul to roam. I mean, you are just leaving my soul to Rome. I feel like I'm burning, facing evil demons who want to take what is left of me and feed. Their greed never had a place in the kingdom, please do not leave me here alone.

With this disease, I cannot believe what I see, or trust what I hear. I walk by faith, not by sight. As far as the kingdom is concerned, I just have to play it by ear. Here, I have something to the equivalent of great wealth. It is my confidence, as I continue to walk through the valley of the shadow of Death.

(2022)
ABSTRACT

My mind has been stretched and twisted to the point of no return. The joy that fills the soul, I swear I missed it. So now I have to find it, or I will burn. Pieces of me have been detached from my body and scattered across the midnight sky. Too abstract to be pieced back together, I yearn to be right, but I do not know why.

Abstractions have hidden secrets, some determining life or death. Still, I write to learn about myself and soul and hope to earn a living until I have retrieved it and obtained substantial wealth. My life one day, I will seize control. Some send their praises to him when they get it. I might snap and say, "What took you so goddamn long to give it?" Look at all I have lost. I have nothing left, too much pain, too much death. Forgive me, these are the thoughts of a schizophrenic. I don't understand how I can praise you one minute and then in the next be ready to knock the heavens and earth down. I guess you teased me with that vision one too many times, in my mind I rewind the vision and make that decision for all my kind. So, I can hear them make that sound.

I load my mind with the clip and blaspheme several rounds. I blast for me, and you too as hot fire enters her mind and exits my mouth. Now we will invade the holy city because the land was ours in the first. Let's take back our city and destroy their king who hath no life. Heaven, my Mahogany, I can see my future with you, because I met you in a past life. Only bloodshed can reverse the curse, cleanse the land, and bring peace to this abstract universe. That is the administration of my last wife. My people, listen to me, what if the one you thought was the evil one was really the good one? And the one you thought was the good one was really evil. How then would you mount your attack? This is how I see the world, people; my perception is hard to be equal because it's just a bit too abstract.

(2022)
BEFORE YOU CAN BLINK TWICE
(A MESSAGE TO WHITE SUPREMACY)

We are the morning star's light residing in dark space inside the midnight. We are forever bonded by melanin's might. You may seek the truth, but you fear what is right.

Look inside of you and you will have a divine insight, and then gifts will be given unto you before you can even blink twice.

Before we could blink twice, our ancestors knew how quickly the world grew and how fast the universe expanded. Within a blink of an eye, everything was in existence. It became so reminiscent of the rate of speed of how everything came to be, the vision that came to me. I could not quite understand it. I think this is how they planned it. It is to be full of mystery, just as the conscience of you and me. We cannot be controlled or corralled because our will is free. Our loyalty, they try to demand it, but we can command our royalty.

Freedom is like striking oil to me, black gold. Our souls are free from those chains of low self-esteem, racism, and bigotry. Now as I pull this intellectual trigger and expose your thoughts to be, before you can blink twice you will think about the word "nigger" and all that you tried to do to us, and you'll see. I can tell we are everything that you want to be, strong, confident, and regenerative.

Before you can blink twice, I can slice the stereotypes and change the narrative. God has the weight of the world on his shoulders and on mine, I am carrying him. So, think twice before you ever disrespect his people because I am them. Because if you do, before you can blink twice, I will show you why you believe we are demonic. We will release an evil so dark you will miss out on the divine spark and be left here for the beast to rip your soul apart, while your loved ones are left wondering. Here is where I will start, with your messiah, the fire is upon him. Zeus cannot be God because we are one of them.

(2022)
OUR MOTHER EARTH:
BEYOND WORDS

As I close my eyes and listen, I see a vision of what I heard; darkness or nothing because of the destruction of our mother earth. Bombs burst replacing bluffing threats with actual deaths lying in the middle of the streets and on the curbs. Countries watch in total shock because a sovereign nation bleeds screaming for peace and wants all of US to intervene to stop the hurt.

To say the least, it is said that creation began with a spoken word. What we are witnessing now we can't speak. Evil is trying to reach its peak. This shit I am seeing is really beyond hope and beyond wordz. I could write a piece begging for peace. But will anybody listen to what it is that I have to say? I pray for better days when we could be released from inside the belly of the beast, onto a higher intelligence to increase the need for love and peace. I asked God to show me the way.

It is beauty that I see today, sunsets at the golden time. I stargaze and activate the melanin from within my mind. As the leaves on the tree speak when there is a breeze saying to me there is more to us than what meets the eye.

I am beholding the beauty of the earth and all of its dimensions; I can now appreciate it for what it's worth. The sea, the moon, the stars, the sun. I am one, speechless as I am encapturing the beauty, really these visions are beyond wordz. I reach out and grab love, before she passes me by. We make contact and I thank the Lord above for bringing her my way, she is the epitome of the Holy Spirit and together we are divine. Her beautiful, Mahogany flesh and Heavenly spirit are mine, and my soul is hers. I am captivated by what you have done for me, I am so blessed, I am truly beyond wordz.

(2022)
GUIDED BY VOICES

I continue to walk in the darkness in pursuit of something that I cannot see. I cannot believe how loud the noise is. Screaming voices are guiding my path through what I believe. It seems that I can feel shapes and objects without being able to see the true reason why I am lost in all this. I see a light at the end flashing, I move closer, and there is a voice asking, "Tim, do you remember me?" I say yes without asking, who you are and how do you know me? I was mesmerized by the lights flashing. I was dashing to get to that, the end, my destiny. All that I had to do was when I felt them, make the right choices, and when within their presence, I just had to be me. Just be guided by their voices until I reach their souls, which ultimately, in the end their essence belongs to me.

From the slightest touch of what they heard, smelled, and tasted, that was so divine. They saw their five senses leave their bodies and with their minds, they became intertwined, with the light of the Father and the heat of the son (sun) and the other heavenly bodies. Really, though, it was just time; this was harder, a harder thing to do, and that is to leave none behind. So, as I listen to you, I continue to speak to me, feeling my way around in the dark until I hit the switch, and I can see what speaks. It was you, Lord, showing me wealth that I am rich, beating with the devil's heart. Your blood flows into my mind. Now knowing that you two are just one of a kind. Let me take a voyage through your souls and mine as I am guided by those voices, until I go past my time.

(2022)
MAKE THE DEVIL PREY

Make the devil prey, as if you starved to be filled with the truth. It is hidden inside the darkness, but your third eyesight is keen, and the true king can see straight through.

I make the devil prey because there is nothing else left to do or feed on. The wealth of heaven has fallen to hell, our earth. I can see 'em moving through the dark, I cast a spell until there is nothing left in you, nothing left to lean on. My instincts and senses are heightened and sparked; no power is withheld.

I began to see through the lies, in which it hides what is really in their hearts, the demons. Believe 'em. I am the lion that ripped them all apart. And then damned them all to hell.

Now that they have been separated from the organic, and everything that constitutes GOD. I prey on 'em at night though understanding that they will never be welcomed back or have the advantage into the depths of Heaven's heart. I prey on the souls and flesh that gave us no rest while we built this nation's body. Chasing freedom without hope for the best, believing in a god whose true intention was to keep us at work with little rest and to keep our families divided.

They were destined to make us slaves, beating and bruising our bodies, until they fell apart, and that part is how they would convince us that we were saved. Jezeus was the noose that hung us from the family tree of our truths and what our ancestors taught. Before they took secrets to the graves, we were made proof that God existed in us, and it was only us in his heart. The chosen ones were saved. I make the devil prey, because that is the only way to feed the beast, who transformed to the greatest from the least once he was filled from the failures of his enemies, now filled with joy plentifully, the carcass of life has him full of vigor and because of that he prays.

I make the devil prey when he refers to me by words, like calling me nigger. When I get em in my sights, I load my mind like a clip, open my mouth, and pull the trigger, to rest their minds.

Kill 'em with words. As soon as I heard the word, I had to eat. It was the only way to bring peace, from within me. My hunger for knowledge had to be fed, it was void and only in one way, taking ownership in my ego, lord of all lords, and making the devil pray, that is the reason why my pride followed me there, because that is where they were led, to a place where I am everywhere. If you pray, why worry? If you worry, why prey? That's what my father said. So, make the devil prey, because if you don't, it just may be your blood that is shed.

(2022)
MY MAHOGANY BYRD

I now realize why I am alive. When you spread those wings, my dream is to show you why. As you took flight, really, it came as no surprise, I was captivated by your presence. Which I know now is the essence of life. It surrounds me and everything that I care to be. To be with you in this way is a privilege, together we are blessed beyond capacity. For my love for you is just a remnant of what our god could be. Even in his infinity that is still not long enough for you and me. I may not as of right now be what you want me to be. But I pray a lot, that now I am right where you need me to be and that is home.

As you have flown me and my family from one end of heaven unto the next. I have shown that to own the present you let go of the past and reach for the future because that comes first and then comes the rest. If you can follow that, then let me lead you into a place in heaven where no soul or angel knows. To the center of our Lord's being, his heart, beating to the beat of the harmony between us. It's all power and music wrapped up intertwining together as one flesh, one soul. For we provide the light, no need for the sun, moon, or stars. Our love glows bright showing the way for lost, damaged, and broken hearts. I don't know where this came from, it was something that, in my head, I just heard. I thank you for flying me to my destination, your imagination, I love you, my Mahogany Byrd.

(2022)
NOT ZEUS, BUT "I AM"

First, let it be known, that the art of not fighting back or taking a passive non-violent approach is derived from the religion of Christianity. They used a white messiah of Rome, JeZEUS (Jesus), as the symbol of white supremacy and it was given to you by your oppressor to keep you feeling inferior. The letter "J" did not exist in any language until over 500 years ago. Around that time, the Spaniards and Portuguese, the Dutch and the British became the first Europeans to participate in the Transatlantic Slave Trade. They worshiped pagan European gods and began bringing Black people to this (Western) region of the planet. Those nations were Zeus worshipers.

Second, let it be known that Zeus, the Roman-Greek King of the Gods, never existed as a physical entity, being, or man. But being that I, like the universe, am black that deep black fact will state that Black lives do matter, and we are the most high and most important part of God's plan. Even in the formation of our universe and in that I can say "I AM," that I am as in the great I am, the Amen, in the flesh as a Black man with life and consciousness. The Hamashiah, or

Messiah, or Ham which means black, or Lord Ham, the anointed one, son of Noaham or Noah. We are higher, higher than the God that they say is king, and what they try to show us. We are Cush Ethiopia, the dream fam, and you too can be as strong as us, and as strong as I Am.

Third, let it be known that everything that the scripture says that belongs to him, is ours strictly because of that lie. It is for us to take. Who among you all are with me? Let us take our proper place. We will devour wealth beyond wealth, power beyond power, and grace beyond grace. Everything that the Heavens are, is us and belongs to us, the richest secrets of the universe. Let us untangle them in their face. As we retrieve the blessings, regardless of love or lust we still feel good, because it is our destiny to be kings and queens of this universe, time, energy, matter, and space redeeming our race… in that, I believe. In that, I trust because our Atom, or Adam was created from cosmic dust. To the imitators and fakes, I say, be damned, now I can honestly say when they ask; "Who is King of Kings and Lord of Lords? Who is the morning star?" Not Zeus, but I AM.

(2023)
HEAVEN ON EARTH

Heaven on Earth, where love and lust meet. Thrusted and intertwined, and connected to form a trust that allows them to fall into a pit that is bottomless. Screamin and hollerin, in my mind I am connected. I hear them as they make everything follow them, yeah, we are fallin that deep.

Into the abyss we sink, as we think of what could possibly be, on the verge of being at the brink, and at the edge of existence, entering & creating another reality. Escaping the former entrapments of this universe, and all of its physicalities, we circle back to before the sexual Big Bang. Back to when we were all virgins, married through thought, love and spirit. Before lust took the form of the physical and made us slaves to beauty, whether physical or through our spirituality, we have become too vain, slaves to a feeling; that feeling becomes our mentality, some are driven insane.

Now I talk to Heaven when I get high, but how high do I have to be? Why would I have to die just to see the true destiny? Instead of bringing me to the sky, I bring the sky to me, where there is no concept of time, no concept of distance, no separation from one point to the next; everything will be within our reach. From the riches and love of Heaven to the beauty and lust of the Earth and vice versa. It's like magic when we think of the seven, a product of the first six, until now I did not understand their worth.

This is Heaven on Earth as I disconnected from everything outside of me, I reconnected with everything within me, the souls of men are many, like the stars and rotating galaxies. I release them from within, bringing God and the universe to the Earth, in the form of two women, and one man. It's a celestial entanglement, as we are connected to everything in a cerebral web of consciousness.

This is a special relationship and arrangement. Just enjoy the pleasure and the truth that comes from it. We now know where we come from, and because of that, if you believe in God, then you know that the future is present, and that is something that we are not far from. Heaven on Earth, this is God and Lucifer united. The Black Man and Black Woman are the essence and importance of creation, a union that cannot be divided. To my enemies and that pale messiah, we are higher than your highness. You watered down the truth about our universe, which is us. Now you must trust and check the science.

This scripture says that the war is already won, it was won once I realized this. That this universe and physical creation is nothing more than an eternal marriage between energy and matter. The stars and space, man, and woman. Even in the hereafter we together in love are amazing grace, and in that way, our lives matter. We live, we die, and then we are rebirthed, and born again with new wisdom, new knowledge, a new life, a new being creating our Heaven on Earth over and over, again and again.

(2023)
INTERNAL WEALTH,
EXTERNAL WEALTH

Which is it that consumes us? Our financial lust can be viewed from two perspectives. Either we work and make it our objective to obtain wealth because we need to feed and satisfy what comes from within; then again, the ego is what conceived the embryo. So, do we have the need to create the best environment so our seed can grow? The next generation wants to make a living. So, do we reap what we sow when our seed has grown and realize that the world is his own and so he takes it, not knowing that the price for that was his soul?

I always thought that killing yourself was the unforgivable sin, at least that's how the story goes. Who are we to pretend that we don't live and work to strive and make money? Either we are working for our families, for ourselves, or to impress our honey. Internal wealth is not only the spiritual wealth within the soul but also that same wealth manifested in the physical outside of the soul. As expected, this notion may not have been reflected. But we live within a body that lives within a body. And so, the view of wealth varies because of our own perspective.

One may wonder about the gold, jewels, and riches of the kingdom of the heavens or the universe. But is this really different in value of the riches that we have here on our planet Earth? Both worlds produce enormous wealth. In a way we have to die to see both. Either you lose your soul and die spiritually for worldly possessions, material wealth, or you die physically to feel and see divine obsessions; or spiritual wealth, heading to a world in which you do not know? One may look at the fact that I have four daughters and may think I have family wealth, but I have lost four aunts to this enemy named death. It was a heavy price to pay to attain spiritual and financial depth. Is there anything else?

I am beyond what is within me. I am now what's outside of me. So how can you judge me on the count of my wealth? My soul, I reside here on earth, but my flesh is beyond my soul. The riches of the soul in the heavens become the riches of the flesh here on earth. The urge to have worth comes from beauty. We are attracted to the beauty. No matter whether it's internal or external. It glitters and glows. The roots of the tree. Scripture says as above, so below. We are valuable to God and to what is above because what is above is valuable to what is below. I am not insane for wanting the riches of the world here on the earth. I am insane because I need the riches and the spirits and souls of the heavens, my true value, my worth.

True gold is an abundance of knowledge and wisdom which you can use to get you into the best financial, and spiritual health and position, a place where you and I can intertwine our visions. Those two worlds - Internal and external wealth - I see it like a premonition. This poem was an attempt to unite science and religion. I am showcasing how the love and lusts of the riches of the heavens or universe, and our souls are in correlation with the loves and lusts of the earth and worldly possessions of the flesh. Scripture says no man can serve two masters.

One would be envious of the other's position. I say they can if the two are made one. Holding the balance is the test that can and will happen, the beautiful caption is the dark of space and the light of the sun, the yin and the yang, the union of man and woman in that birth in all religions. And in that and from that, wealth happens, and then we become conditioned.

(2023)
TRUE IGNORANCE:
WHO ARE WE? WHO ARE YOU?

This Piece Is Addressed to Claims of Anti-Semitism. Not that I aim to offend anyone, but a lot of you have offended me. Being that everyone and everything is derived from one source, this piece of art, and it is art, was meant to shed light on a subject in which the people who look like me, have succumbed unto great and terrible scrutiny for trying to discover something that has been taken from them (us) as a people. With that said, you have the likes of old racist, negative, and imposing political figures, who can make statements about the Jews of Israel as compared to the Jews of America and still be able to proceed with their agenda without financial or critical backlash or suffering of any consequences for this ignorance. TRUE IGNORANCE. So, if Black people are not the true people of God, being that everyone derived from one source, then I ask you... *Who Are We? Who Are You?*

(2022)
WHO ARE WE? WHO ARE YOU?

Ask yourself, do you know who you are, who you really are? If you do, then you will be able to accept this. First, I want to start with this. How can anyone black be antisemitic, when the origins of Judaism and Christianity began with Black people? You need to just accept it.

The true evil is that most non-Melanated people hate the fact that we are superior within the entity, meaning, we are where the energy has been entrapped and so their focus is on us. So, in that way, we are the only way back. Do you know you? Do you know what makes you Hebrew? No bar mitzvah or any man-made tradition in your religion can make you true.

I will ask you again, "Do you know what makes you Hebrew?" Check the verses in Leviticus 46 and Deuteronomy 28 in the Old Testament scripture, then you will know if this race of people is you. It has nothing to do with the six million people dying in concentration camps but has everything to do with hundreds upon hundreds of millions of Black people murdered for over a millennium due to the hands of racism and the Transatlantic Slave Trade; Masters branding our people with their stamps as if we are their property. Hell, we were their property, as displayed.

I want to save those who prayed. Now it ain't no stopping me, if you as a race of people are not suffering from those curses listed in the verses above, well then you are not the chosen ones of God. True Israel is suffering, lost, and torn apart cursed with poverty and death throughout their history not ready to receive the Father's love. So, if you are Jewish and you are wealthy, how could you have God's heart? Jews are among some of the richest people on the planet. Dammit, they have had their reparations, what have Black people received for playing their part. The truth of the matter is that every other race on the planet has generated over a trillion dollars off of Black people, and we as a people have not benefited at all from this, we are treated as if we are less than equal. Lord, free us from this evil.

Most of the people who say they are the true Jews are imposters. Residing in the land promised to us by God, originally occupied by our forefathers. True Israel is spread out to the four corners of the earth, suffering collectively as a race of people because of a God given evil curse. What's worse is that most Black people are so lost that they don't even know why.

But it's because we worship pagan gods and idols and partake in pagan religious practices, even though most know that those religions are a lie. Who are we, a people with a lost identity? The time it is said that the Hebrews spent in Egypt is said to be a metaphor for Blacks to realize who they are, and to be brought back to prominence and have resources restored back plentifully. To the Jewish community, I ask you, who are you, if you are not the true people of God? Who are you worshiping in your synagogues if you don't believe that a Messiah walked? We as Black people make up the body of the Lord, matter, and the stars.

Call it the Christ, for the crystallization of the stars. No one can come unto the father unless they go through the son (sun) we are the light, and we are the lord and light in everyone. Most Jews believe that they are in the truth without any evidence or any real proof. How do you believe these things if you know you infiltrated the African religions after Israel fell to Rome in 70 A.D. and then proceeded to breed and intermix the races and also mix religions until we have what we see today; Inside of the holy land, European people claiming that they are the subject of racism, bigotry, and hate, but I say there is only one truth born from one group. We are the original people on the planet. Now, I ask you again and hope that you have an understanding, *who are we?* Or better yet, *who are you?*

(2023)
IF I COME UP, YOU COME DOWN

Blessings. I can point out millions of them in the span of a day. Some people, though, are pessimistic and negative. Interfering with the ascension in detention because of a disease called jealousy and envy, where you hate plenty, every day, all day. The dissension and descending are blessings from the most high; that's why, when I come up, you come down, when I am most high. Blessings from here to bling town in Heaven, they can be found. I would not lie.

I write about my thoughts and feelings inside of me, they have been circling forever; my mind goes, merry, go round, I'm dizzy inside. Cycling like planets, stars, and galaxies, amazed, I drop to my knees, worrying, and I pray. Then I ask God for his amazing immaculance, if I come up, will you come down, flourishing? Blessings. If I come up, best believe they are going to come down.

For all of my people who work increasingly hard for a little bit of nothing, not quite enough, retrieving wealth, so those who have worked can play. It seems to be the only way now. Before I die, I want to know what it's like to spend $1 million. Before I die, I want to know what it's like to give someone $100 million. All of this, just so I can make your soul holler. Louder than the ones burning in the depths of hell, you can't tell, I need your souls on full throttle. So, one day we can sit back, relax with our riches & wealth, and pop champagne bottles. The good life. One day I got to live it up. My good life. One day I will have to give it up. When that day comes, Lord, I will be ready. But if I come up, you come down, with blessings, real heavy.

(2020)
SUNSETS ON SATURN

I can be the one who you dream about at night. You know touchin' your soul with my brain until you quiver and deliver as we are sexually insane. As we attain thought and anticipation of us creamin' together, coming together before the sunset right before I skated through the rings. I entered Saturn's astronomical plane. As I entered Saturn's atmosphere, it was simple and plain.

This domain was filled with love plus a little fear because there is no ground to touch; my feet could not be planted. I swear this was not the way we created this mission and planned it. This planet is too beautiful to not have a solid ground, a foundation so we could build from the ground up. It is colorful, and not because its number was the sixth, but because we know what lives in it.

Rest assured, her beauty is appreciated and adored from her colorful atmosphere to her melanated core, also known as the most high, lord. Oh lord, now this union between us has flourished and become a pattern, and right when I found the light, we see the sun sets on Saturn.

(2023)
THE FASCINATION WITH GREEN

Like something out of a dream, I'm fascinated with you. To be true, I have been infatuated with you. You never knew that in 1996, we would develop a friendship, in which after we first met, learning to drive, I hope that our conversations you would not forget. So, I began experimenting with weed and then wet, hoping to rise to a high to remember the stimulating conversating we used to do. The God in me talking with the Heaven within you made us divine, and in my mind, I rewind our conversations with all the time, you know, as if a song was played, and the rhythm, beat, and melody stayed and then there is the hook, it was your look I couldn't get out of my mind.

It seemed in our senior year we realized that we, you and me, could be onto something here. Both of us were surprised at how special our connection was, and that we both felt like there could be something special about the uniting of us. We never realized that true love for both of us, the fate of it was on borrowed time. You see, soon, we would graduate, and a new life we would create or find. While we were away and on our first year off, I swear I felt and heard you pray because I remembered how you felt about GOD; remembering back I wasn't really that lost. I remember talking.

We expressed to each other on that day when you came to visit me once we were licensed. You came to my house. I believe your admiration was trying to reach through to me, but it was something that I was too busy fighting, and it never got through until a year later when we were home for the summer from school.

And it was then that I felt like the biggest fool. I was suffering. I had the heavens unknowingly on both sides, pulling my soul in a tug-of-war for spiritual existence and dominance. I thought this may be my last and only chance at happiness and prominence. This particular day, I was trying to tell you something. I had something important to say. For whatever reason, the message would not be relayed. There were feelings and voices, telling me to kill myself; the more I tried to reveal, the more they enhanced. You would not understand how deeply and strongly I still cared for you, or how I felt. My thoughts and words began circling and running; running away from you, away from the truth, that I was falling in love with you; but I was dead and in you too. And the truth was that there was no Messiah coming.

Unfortunately for me, this was the beginning of the end of Tim, as we all once knew him. Schizophrenia took over, and I said to the Heavens, and to God, "Be damned, screw them." It seems that the only thing that matters in life is the Green. If I ever get to have you,

I pray that you are pure, natural, potent, and without any seeds. *How many of us spend our lives trying to get it and keep it?* But we never seem to appreciate why we need it. In my case, I need it to grow to survive. Not just for a financial or material high, but because you do something to my soul, for my soul. You are an elevator to Heaven, and that is what I saw in your Mahogany, brown skin, Heaven's eyes underneath that Green, pure gold, and in that is the light that I remember through my dark hour.

The true power lies with the me in you, and you with the you in me. That is what I'm fascinated with, God's soul. You are a light and that makes me whole and makes me want to fight anything for you like the Panther you are. I love you, always, and that now I can roar sincerely yours, and yours truly.

If there is a Messiah, he exists only because of your memory of me and in that we get higher. Do you feel me? If I didn't tell you, I'd be a liar. You are the substance of things hoped for, but the evidence of things unseen. You are like faith; do you know what I mean? This is my fascination with Green.

Dedicated to Lydia Yvonne Green, remember me. -Timothy- The One True King

(2023)
MELANIN

The study of melanin was originally viewed by our European brothers as demonic. Voodoo, witchcraft, sorcery, black magic, telekinesis, shapeshifting, telepathy, and various other crafts dealing with melanin and the mind and of inner-dimensional realms were shunned and frowned upon and kept hidden from Black people once the Transatlantic Slave Trade began sometime between 70 A.D. and the 14th century.

Any knowledge of teachings of these abilities were all but erased in the consciousness of Black people all over the planet. Caucasian people viewed these things as a threat to what they were believing and what they were trying to introduced to the masses of the African people; whom Rome had conquered in 70 A.D. and whom, along with the Spaniards, Portuguese, the Dutch, and the British, then took the masses of the Hebrews (Israelites) and some other African tribes involuntarily, kidnapping them from their tribes and made them slaves.

Now mind you, the best way to conquer and enslave a race of people is to attack their belief systems and religious practices. So, they took the one thing that made us who we are, and they demonized it. They then told us that we shouldn't practice it because it's evil and there is no place for it in the kingdom of God (Heaven).

The truth of the matter is they are telling us not to learn about ourselves, but the kingdom of heaven (the universe) is made up of the very same thing that they have labeled daemonic... Melanin. *Why is that?* I will tell you why; it's simply to hide our identity.

Third Eye Publishing

PART VI

Conclusions

Third Eye Publishing

LIVING WITH SCHIZOPHRENIA

As I stated in my first book, the word Amen produced the word Damien which begat the word demon. The term amen means "What is hidden," our identity is hidden.

The term Amen-RA is also connected to the sun and to the "I am" as in the great "I am." RA is the revealing or what comes to light. The AM Is significant as it means Lord. Even though we are the darkness, and we are actually a part of that demonic labeling, we are on both sides of the table. The term illuminati is derived from Lucifer, it means the light bearer, or being of extraordinary brilliance. Since we are associated with the demonic anyway by the Europeans, we also carry the light. Light is energy. Energy is life. We are the other side, as is the meaning of the word "Hebrew." We are the pioneers of science, mathematics, agriculture, and religion. We civilized the Europeans, brought them out of the darkness of the icy, Caucus Mountains (thus named Caucasians) in which they were living in filth with the animals, and practiced incest and cannibalism, while being entrapped there for thousands of years due to the drastic climate change on the planet. Because of this, their whole physical makeup changed and they went from looking like us, until what we have today. After the great flood that has been documented by so many different cultures, Noah's ark, as said in the book of Genesis, rested on Mt. Arrat in Turkey. Whether you believe this story or not, I must inform you, in case you do not know, that in 1959 a massive boat-like object was discovered from a satellite out in orbit resting on the top of Mt. Arrat. Some 30 years later they realized that the object was wedged inside of the mountain. The Turkish government would not allow anyone from any other countries to excavate and visit the area. But it was soon visited by few excavators that the Turkish government allowed, and they discovered that there were petrified animal droppings inside of the arch. After the flood, the families of Noah (Noham) went in different directions. The family of Ham went back south back to the land of Havaillah or Ethiopia in Northeast Africa. This family consist of Ham the youngest son of Noah (Noham), his son's Cush (Ethiopia), Mizraim (Egypt or Kemmitt), Phut (Libya), and Canaan (land of the Canaanites) all of the African nations are derived from this lineage. Then Shem and his descendants settled east (Arabian Countries, or middle eastern countries) and Japeth (European countries, and Gentile nations) and his descendants traveled and settled north. This is where they would get trapped there for thousands of years, around the time of the ice age. They would undergo a major transformation, losing their skin pigmentation, growth of hair all on their exterior, eye coloration transformation, their bone structure transformed and the most telling of all their pineal gland had become calcified, dormant, and non -

existent. The cold weather became the main factor in their savagery, and why they seem to have the most evil of intent. They were savages and they lived that way until the Black Moors from Morocco came to bring them into the light and teach them science, mathematics, agriculture and our religious practices and spiritual knowledge. Also, child raising, and how to eat the proper way. After, once they learned how to create gun powder from the Chinese, that's when the great takeover began. Before then Black people had the wealth and power.

As for their belief in the kingdom of heaven, which is light, life and brilliance, the only way for them (Gentile nations) to get there is through us. We are the only way into the kingdom of heaven, and unto the Father. We are good and evil, God and Lucifer, positive and negative. Black men are the stars inside our Black women who are the dark matter and space. Together forever, the Black family is the universe.

For 25 years or more, I had all of these things weighing on me. I had countless thoughts of ending my life because I just couldn't find a clear answer. I would pray to God and ask Him why He would place me with this task. There was no clear-cut way of achieving what was placed in my heart. It seemed impossible, but blindly I believed. Racing thoughts would pass before I could get a clear perspective. I was frustrated because at the time, when I was first diagnosed, no one would engage in a conversation about what I was feeling. No one wanted to listen. I had no one to turn to. No one would talk to me about it, so I would just talk to the voices.

Smoking marijuana helped, because when I smoked, the voices would become louder, a bit clearer if you will. In my sober mind, I couldn't quite make out what they were saying. It was like something was in there trying to reach me, but it was not getting through. Just clouded thoughts all jumbled up with no escape. I would smoke and it would open things up and slow my thoughts down. Things began to flow… It made a world of difference. I could clearly hear what the voices were saying, and I also could identify each one while receiving visions from each one. Some were cryptic, some were apocalyptic, some were divine, some were euphoric and pleasant, and then some were supernatural. I embraced all of these things that the voices were showing me. I wanted more, I craved more… They were teaching me things that I was not going to learn in any church or university. They made a direct correlation linking the Black man and the universe.

Somehow, I became the center of all of it. This especially at that time, with something that Black people could not believe, and some white people would kill you if they heard anyone making the assessment that Blacks are superior.

Still, I became addicted to the knowledge that was being channeled through to me from my family in the heavens. I was addicted to the connection; the ancestors, pre and post enslavement. I had to smoke weed in order to hear them clearly, otherwise all I would just hear was a bunch of unorganized noise in my head. That is the curse of Schizophrenia. For years, I spent my time and energy trying to make out what the voices were trying to say and trying to get others to see what I was seeing. I guess that is the very thing that makes us unique. It is also the very thing that causes many of the people who suffer from this disease to do the unthinkable... commit suicide.

So, I guess my mission with this, my second publication, is to try and provide an avenue or avenues that shed light on why people like me eventually suffer the ultimate fate.

Living with Schizophrenia can be a very detrimental hindrance to those closely related to the individual, or the individuals themselves. Many of those afflicted cannot be productive because many of them do not realize that they are gifted. One of the best coping mechanisms when dealing with Schizophrenia is realizing your creativity as it relates to your importance, and the importance of utilizing your talents and gifts as it relates to your mental condition.

It is imperative to find things to be positive about, which you can utilize as a weapon or weapons to keep pushing positive-thinking against a somewhat warped thought-pattern that comes with having this illness. Just feeling good about something, even if it is something minor, can make all of the difference when someone is contemplating whether to continue to live or not. You have to have something or someone to want to live for, even if that means finding success in trivial things to generate some sense of joy and accomplishment. You have to take baby steps first, depending on the severity of the condition.

You will have good days and bad days, but the most important thing is that you learn from each passing day, and what you learn you can capitalize on future days. In my case, future days could mean more tragedy. Let me explain why I struggle with taking my medication.

No one should attach themselves to my situation because everyone's situation and mental state are different. When I first met my psychiatrist, we had a conversation about my voices. I told her that the voices that I hear inside my head are too strong to destroy because they are my family members. This was in 1999 around the time I was first diagnosed. I told her that the connection was too strong and that she would not be able to break the attachment. In her words, she said, "Watch me."

So, two years later the first of the voices, the first angel, that I heard was my Uncle Larry, he died in a freakish accident. That was in 2001. In 2010, another voice that was in my head became silenced after another freak accident that took place on a luxury cruise. This was my Aunt Rita, who suddenly drowned in the waters of Cozumel, Mexico. She was the fourth angel and voice in my head.

Uncle Larry and Aunt Rita were my mother's oldest brother and little sister who suffered those fates. Later on, that year in 2010, another one of the seven voices was silenced, as my mother's closest sister, my Aunt Cheryl passed away from cancer. This was the third angel and voice in my head preceding the death of my grandfather in 2017, who was the father of the six people and the grandfather of the seventh who was already inside of my mind. In 2018 the sixth angel and voice inside of my mind had suddenly grown ill and died of kidney failure. This was my mom's youngest Brother, Uncle Gregory, or G.

And now, just as I continue to write and create my second book, I am saddened once again. The seventh and most important and loudest voice in my head, my oldest cousin, the seventh angel, Latroy, was now gone from a heart attack as of October 14, 2022. I can't begin to tell you what I am and have been going through. I figured out what I thought was a connection to the voices that, actually, started dying off. It was the medication.

The medication altered my focus from them to my doctor. I figured that the medication has some kind of deadly kinetic connection with the people whom I admire the most by rearranging where I sent my energy. My doctor said she would destroy them all, and I'll just be damned if she isn't doing it... one by one.

Now there are just two left physically and they are at war right now with each other. My mother and her baby sister. The second and fifth angels. It certainly seems as if there is a connection there between the medication, the seven voices, and my seven family members. This is the main reason why I struggle to take the medicine. Not only because of the loss of life but also because the medication suppresses what is trying to come out. So, the only way to bring it out of me in a peaceful way is to write about it.

Still though, I find it hard to express exactly how and what is happening to me. Hundreds and hundreds of millions of Black people throughout the Transatlantic Slave Trade lost their lives because they were just being themselves. Lots of them were raped, murdered, and separated from their families. Why, because they were expressing who God was, just by living their lives as queens and kings. In every way, their emotions were suppressed and oppressed by the very thing that is suppressing my thought process and spiritual growth.

The European influence from the medicine used to treat mental illness to the educational institutions to the religious institutions to the economic and financial system with their main goal being to control, conquer, and divide. Now with this "critical race theory" wanting to omit the teachings about slavery and pre-enslavement, Black history in schools to the upcoming generation is another attempt to cover up their evil and barbaric behavior, and heinous crimes.

One white Florida politician labeled it (pre-enslavement Black history) dangerous. It's hard to believe that with 85% of the people on this planet being Black or people of color we can't seem to come together, organize, and mobilize, and completely transform the state of the original people and their planet. If we took every Black billionaire on the planet (in which there are 15) and if each one of them gave a substantial amount to poverty-stricken areas in their communities and even other poverty-stricken communities, we could change the landscape and narrative that we have to depend on our respective governments for assistance. Even if they were just involved in their communities, sharing their knowledge on how they obtained their wealth and how others could do the same would be very beneficial to the state of mind of a broken people relying on a broken system.

Give them avenues that they can take to steer them in the correct direction until they can manifest a lucrative financial opportunity for themselves. You change the mind state of the people in the community, then you change the state of the community. With just 15 Black billionaires worldwide, if each one produced three more billionaires it would become forty-five and it would just keep multiplying. That's one way you could swing the pendulum back in our direction, provided that each Black billionaire does the right thing.

ACCOLADES TO MY FAMILY

My roots stay pure, and my values and loyalty lie with my mother and father; of course, my mother, the one who brought me into this world, I will always be loyal to and love religiously. But it was my father, whose voice was silent in my mind, but present when I spoke my words of truth and righteousness. It was he who created me and sacrificed so my sister and I could have a good life.

My father is the reason I'm able to balance and keep it together. It was he who channeled his prayers and energy into my mind so that when I would function and operate, I would do so with his commands all through my physical and spiritual being. He is the head of the lion, and I am the body. Though I struggle with all of these issues that I have described to you over the course of these two books I have written, I have never meant for my own personal struggles to affect my beautiful sister, wife, and children.

To them, I want to say that I apologize for it all. All of it. To Mahogany, my sister, and my niece, I never meant to inflict them with the pain that I felt. To my children, niece, and nephews, I just want you to know that I love you more than the air that I breathe.

You are that valuable to me, I need to see your dreams come true. It is the main motivation for why I write. I write so that I can provide a financial avenue for you all to go after your life's passion.

My eldest child, I always taught you to look within yourself for the answers to the mysteries of the universe. Also, I taught you the meaning of your Blackness and why it is so important to hold true to your core values and to remember who you are.

To my second child, I always taught you that you can think yourself out of any situation, whether it be internal or external. You can outthink any opposition. I also taught you that we as a people already know everything. We just have to remember.

My third child. You have my heart, and I always taught you that God and your lost loved ones are always here with you and when you are troubled, I taught you to pray.

Finally, my youngest, Nadia, the world has yet to get wind of you but when they do, it will be like "Whoa, Kemosabe!" in the name of your Sabby. Look, this universe is art to me, and all of its beauty and chaos has been painted inside of my mind. So, for that reason alone, I want to try and bring what is inside out. I don't claim to be the smartest or most educated person in the world, but what I have found is really quite simple, if you think about it.

There is Father God, then there is Mother Nature, and then there is us. With my situation with Mahogany and Heaven, I'm trying to show the world that I have manifested the very skepticism about God the Almighty, into a real-life reality and now anything is possible if you know of the things that I have articulated in these two books.

We are not many, we are one. Many are called, but only a few are chosen. Those few are the ones who understand that we have a spiritual father and spiritual mother, and thus we have life. So, with that life, I give you more of my life. Hey, I just played the cards that I was dealt. For so long, I was the subject of ridicule and bullying because I was different. People didn't understand me. Hell, I couldn't understand myself. However, I yearned for Heaven, to me she was the epitome of knowledge and wisdom, and that is what I wanted, what I needed. I just didn't know that it would come in the form of a woman.

Both of the Heavens and Mahogany represented everything good to me and they all were once within my reach to be molded into pure gold by me, and not fools' gold. I just used what I had within my reach to grab what was really important, and that turned out to be us. All of us. The whole race of people. This is also the soul of the Heavens and the Mahogany Earth. That means more to me than anything else. I want the souls to dance to the beat of my heart, because that's what I write to. Life is harmonic balance, meaning everything is done in rhythm. It is the beauty of the stars and space, energy and material, consciousness and matter, man and woman, God and Goddess.

I will continue to prove that the Big Bang was a sexual play between a man and a woman. It just proves that this universe was born out of love. Just as the vagina contracts and expands, so does this universe. We are 13.8 billion years in its expansion and for me, I'm waiting to go back in so we can explode out again. Life is a marriage (Revelations 19 and 21), and a marriage takes work by both parties to CREATE a life. We are that life.

(2023)
MY SOUL IS ON FIRE

I'm burning, not because I am evil, but because I am so obsessed and in love with the Heavens, I turned on my people. My people, well, me and my people shall I say. I pray that if Heaven is for real, my heart will heal. It was broken in two because of what I revealed to you, the two that gave me a way. But still, there was one in which held my true heart's desire. I tried to make it back to her, before my father threw her to the demons, which would give me a reason to jump headfirst into the fire. Without thinking and seemingly controlled by something other than me, I acted and dove right in, without checking to see if I belonged there, checking to see if I was with or without sin.

It is said that Hell is the truth seen too late, and that Heaven has to be brought out from within. I remember her oh so long ago, her light was my energy emitted from my people's soul. Whom I said I would not forsake. Seven of them, each one of them representing a billion souls, they were the light, and that light was for her sake. The light clothed the body and flesh of Heaven, and the light was with men, and that's where it all began.

You see, I had a hallucinogenic vision that my dear Heaven was burning, no longer pure and clean, the light that she possessed drew lustful men to her, and with her they wanted to be filthy and unclean. The vision came to me when I was just nineteen. Around the time I read Revelations, Chapter19, and realized that this girl was my dream. I knew that to make her clean and ask God for her hand, I would have to make a sacrifice, one like no other man. So, I offered up my soul to be damned to the pits of Hell, fire, and brimstone only if you, Father, would relieve her of a lustful spell of sex, violence, and lies, and exchange her soul for mine, and bring her back home.

Where she belongs, is with my flesh, and in Heaven, the other side, the other one, because now it is my soul that is burning forever. Why, you might ask, because I sacrificed my character by exploring my lustful desires to make sure that the integrity and character of Heaven is pure and intact so that the city is protected in a way that's so clever, we are near. To lust is to burn. And now my body and being are craving Heaven in the worst way. I am burning because my people, those 7 angels, those 7 billion, would not recognize my love for them and Heaven, and so to the Heavens, I turn my back away. It is the true definition of what love is, for one to spiritually die for another to physically live.

Whether you believe in me, or Heaven, at this point, I don't think it really matters, but that is what I did for you. I died and cried in my lust, just so you can experience life, love, and laughter here, in the hereafter, we are the closest thing to God, and then that I trust.

As for my people, I did what I should, in hopes of bringing you back as close to the kingdom of Heaven as I could. If I had never expressed my true love for Heaven, then I would have truly been a deceiver and a liar. But because I challenge God and everything that love stands for in my lust over my true love that I wanted forever, somehow a believer's soul was set on fire.

About the Author

Timothy V. Lane

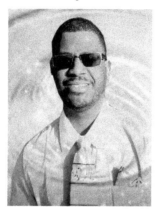

I have Schizophrenia, which is an imbalance of chemicals in the brain, naturally for me. I am out of order with the laws of the natural Universe (which would explain why some still say schizophrenia is demonic). I think differently from most. Some say I think backwards which may explain why I am so set on the creator and creation and where we come from, because wiser men have said you can't know where you are going unless you know where you come from.

CHANNELING THE WHISPERS WITHIN: a Schizophrenic's Journey Through the Labyrinth of Life is my Second published book. My first published book is ***TRAPPED INSIDE MY MIND: 7 Dimensions in Black and White; Poetry from the Perspective of a Schizophrenic.***

Printed in the USA
CPSIA information can be obtained
at www.ICGtesting.com
JSHW060959220324
59547JS00003B/6